# COMING HOME

Coping With a Sister's Terminal Illness
Through Home Hospice Care

# COMING
# HOME

Coping With a Sister's Terminal Illness
Through Home Hospice Care

Cynthia Pincus Russell, PhD

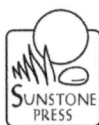

SUNSTONE
PRESS

SANTA FE

Sunstone books may be purchased for educational, business, or sales promotional use.
For information please write: Special Markets Department, Sunstone Press,
P.O. Box 2321, Santa Fe, New Mexico 87504-2321.

Book and Cover design ›Vicki Ahl
Body typeface › California FB
Printed on acid-free paper
∞

Library of Congress Cataloging-in-Publication Data

Russell, Cynthia Pincus, 1935-
  Coming home : coping with a sister's terminal illness through home hospice
care / by Cynthia Pincus Russell.
    p. cm.
  Includes bibliographical references.
  ISBN 978-0-86534-874-5 (softcover : alk. paper)
1. Deery, Diantha Fitch, 1932---Health. 2.  Terminally ill--Biography.
3. Terminally ill--Care. 4.  Critical care medicine. 5.  Hospice care. I. Title.
R726.8.R87 2012
362.17'5092--dc23
[B]
                              2012002720

**WWW.SUNSTONEPRESS.COM**
SUNSTONE PRESS / POST OFFICE BOX 2321 / SANTA FE, NM 87504-2321 /USA
(505) 988-4418 / ORDERS ONLY (800) 243-5644 / FAX (505) 988-1025

Dedicated to my grandparents
Sterling and Rebecca
who left me their home
and their spirit!

# CONTENTS

# INTRODUCTION

You're returning from a conference at the other end of the country, switch on the answering machine at two in the morning, and hear the words "I'm dying." First, of course, you know it can't be true. But this time it is.

What is it like to find out that someone you love is terminally ill and has less than two months? And how do you drop everything to create an instant Home Hospice?

I had often thought that I would likely take in my sister, someday, in old age, to live with me. I was ready to become her care giver, as she had been mine when we were children. That was one reason for moving back into the family's 1790 "Homestead"—an ideal place to take in any relative or friend with all its many rooms. When I was a girl, these rooms were full of relatives, a cousin in need of better schooling, a widowed great uncle, a war bride, baby and GI husband living off the kitchen right after World War II.

But that was years in the future: we were young and vigorous, weren't we? What made it especially shocking were her energy and seeming health; a 64-year-old, living independently in the country with her animals, doing all her own chores, baking her own bread and cookies, a "health person" knowing every remedy and all manner of country things. Six weeks elapsed from diagnosis to death.

I write about process: laughter one moment over an old recording of Nichols and May on the ever-talking radio in the corner of her room; calling the doctor the next over a sudden, alarming symptom, helping her climb onto a chair to spray a wasp's nest on the back porch, seeing the blood-red ambulance pull into the drive. I deal with the experience of caring for my only sister, my only remaining relative of my age and the generation before, mother, father, aunts and uncles. With letting go of my life, with no family to support me in the area where we live to support me through the days and nights of suspense, so that she can let go as easily as possible. To never know what lies around the next corner: blood, pain, an inability to catch a breath, and how one can get through it. About listening twenty-four hours a day for a faint voice calling from a room down the hall, a beep on my cell phone.

My purpose is to help others. To know the incredible strength that lies within us all when we know how to call on it. To juggle the two separate lives of working while caregiving for someone with many requests and needs, caused by the body and emotions of a person approaching their exit. To handle the particular challenge of all of this when you are a rescuer by nature, or a professional caregiver used to putting the needs of everyone else first, without falling on your face from imbalance.

Sharing philosophies and strategies comes naturally to me as a Psychosynthesist. Much of my learning comes out of this system of recovery and growth developed by the Italian psychiatrist Roberto Assagioli. This deep respect for the client-patient is also profound in the work of Bernie Siegel, MD[1] for whose agency I have been health professionals' trainer, teaching conscious dying and how to lead groups for people with cancer, AIDS and other show-stopping diagnoses. Years before today's new field of psychoneuroimmunology, researching the immune response and survival, Bernie knew and taught intuitively that hope can be life-supporting. Now it was my turn to walk as a human being through the valley of the shadow of death in which I had been guiding others as a counselor.

# PRELUDE

Since the age of five, I have been intrigued with things medical. My earliest impressions were filled with the awe we had for our father, a neurosurgeon, who would go off to operate at dawn, and saved hundreds of lives by mysterious weavings of nerves and vessels in the wee hours.

When I was in grade school, he once brought home watercolors done by a child patient and displayed them in the well of Mother's dressing table mirrors in the hall. I was down with the flu, but vividly remember standing in front of them, fever and all—longing to become a child painter who could impress him too. He was as distant as the moon in my life. If you were sick, he might come and sit on your bed for a few moments. Otherwise he was far, far, away.

At night, sometimes my big sister and I were permitted at the grown-up supper table with him and my mother and allowed to listen to stories of patients and hospitals, setting the stage for my lifelong involvement with them.

For the past ten years, I've been doing research on patient experiences, inspired by a huge document, *Iatrogenicity in a large medical center*, which appeared mysteriously on my desk when I'd landed a new job in a huge hospital. When they had no cases for me the first few days, I had, of course, karmically speaking, to read the thing cover to cover. A medical resident's thesis became a mission and purpose for me. Many cases of my own have since led me to a deeper and deeper conviction that these were important stories and must not be forgotten.

My sister took a different path and volunteered in the veterans' hospital where she saw vets in pain, vets neglected, even vets with cigarettes burning their lips, with no one there to remove them. She was inspired to bring them plants and home-baked cookies, fish, and baby chicks—anything that spoke of life. (This was years before the world caught on to the plant and pet therapies of today!)

In recent years, I'd been asked to teach for Bernie Siegel and was immersed in hope and healing and even 'conscious dying' in my workshops, which had opened new windows into living. Dee kept scrapbooks on illnesses and remedies, was known as "the health person" in our family, and we always had so much to talk about! Like those twins separated at birth studied in research recently, who have the same hobbies, name their children the same names, and buy the same cars. Dee and I sprang from the same gene pool, giving meaning to our lives in random patterns, like Jackson Pollack spattering paint drops onto canvases.

I should know about crisis; I have been counseling people for more than three decades. Yet there is something so totally overwhelming about a true crisis that words fail. I experienced this first when I was told my father had died as a child, with no preparation, and not having been able to see him, or my family, for over six months. A second taste was when half my house burned in the middle of the night.

"This is a true trauma," the fire chief counseled me. "Very few experience this, but it is a major trauma. Take it easy. Go slow. Call if you need help." So much gratitude welled up in me that I have no idea what I said.

A third time was the bitter taste of terror as my son lay gasping for breath in the hospital, and it had taken me a good five minutes to drag several "code" people out of another room because they had not heard the buzzer.

What can you tell another? That it feels like a gigantic steamroller coming toward you, running over you. A hand, a touch, a hug—all there is room for at first. Find someone to talk to. You will have to. Get yourself a little notebook and write, write, write. What you've done. What you need to do. What you think. One husband (of a woman with a massive brain tumor) called it "Command Central." For me, it was the thread to survival.

This becomes your memory, collects essentials, helps you reorganize, and stores feelings and emotions for later, when you will be longing to harvest them. So much life can be lost in numbness.

Caregivers are overwhelmed partly because the terrain is completely unknown to us. If only someone could give us a map.

If you connect to any form of Higher Power, this is the time to use it. The Norman Vincent Peale Center receives two thousand calls a day now! We do not know the precise mechanism that makes it work, but the power of prayer is becoming well documented in research,[4] as at the Southern California Medical Center where prayer was correlated with fewer complications and symptoms for patients following heart surgery.

My purpose in writing this book is to help others walk the tightrope of working at a fulltime job and caregiving at the same time. The challenge of combining these two tasks is especially overwhelming when you are also a professional caregiver, used to putting everyone else first.

I have divided the book into two sections. The first is a daily journal of how I walked through it and what I learned. The second and shorter part is a collection of thoughts, quotes and references that might be of help to others in a similar situation. I also include a short section on ways to clarify and center.

# PART 1
# THE DAILY JOURNAL

had looked forward to the late summer for over a year. It would be a time when I could finally "let go." Unpack from a very rapid move the year before (the house sold the first day it was on the market). Breathe. Take time to balance other parts of my life after a year packed full of psychotherapy, workshops and teaching. But there was something else I needed to do, and I was about to find out.

## July 28th

Finally entering my bedroom at three in the morning, I switch on my answering machine. There's a message in my sister's voice.

"I'm dying. Aunt N. has had a massive hemorrhagic stroke the same day I found out. Please call me."

Is there any possibility I *wouldn't*? Has the entire older generation of my family been wiped out in one day? For a moment I don't react because she's been a hypochondriac many, many, times; told me she will die, and soon. Is this time *real*?

Trembling, I lie down and let my head sink into the softness of the pillow. Can't call at three in the morning. Maybe if it's true, she's at least getting the relief of sleep. I'm far too wound up to sleep and switch on the radio. A bomb blast at the Olympics. Rock Concert. A heavy sigh comes out of me from somewhere. I can't feel where. I am cold and frightened.

I think back to the Psychosynthesis conference in San Diego, playing with my friends, sneaking off to the carnival that is Venice, Mission Bay. What fun to travel with Isabelle. Yet when she had a "hunch" we should leave a day early, I, too, feel the creepy-crawly of the "truth response" Anne has told me about and agree instantly. It is a shivery sensation. You just *know*.

Flying back, the skies were so clear I felt for the first time as if this country belonged to me. I could see into the brown of the desert, the peaks of the high mountains. On previous trips I was too occupied with the children, or too frightened, to peer straight down. Getting older is accompanied by large doses of bravery. In return, I am given a gift: sunset at the astral level.

Over my shoulder, a fluffy bank of pink clouds developed, grew and grew, and led my gaze through a golden arbor above them and into a sunset as high as heaven. I was literally breathless at this strange and miraculous sign. What might it mean?

Then I curled up, looking forward to just relaxing at home, the end of the summer, unpacking, settling, putting down some roots after my giant, draining move. As we approached JFK, I thought of the bodies in the water from the explosion of TWA 800. Waiting to be located and a story to be told? I prayed for them, and their families.

Sleep finally came. "Knitting up the raveled sleeve of care," as Shakespeare said. How merciful. I hope she slept. First thing, I call her. She answers as one who is sitting on the phone.

"Dee, how dreadful! Are you positive? How do you know for sure?"

"The first doctor hugged me after the exam and told me it was cancer. She didn't think it had spread. The second was so nasty, the surgeon. He said, 'Better just plan on staying in the hospital when you come in for the test. You'll be having surgery.' He was absolutely horrible."

I take a gulp of air, trying to think as fast as I possibly can. "Don't do anything until we get a second opinion. I'm going to call around."

"Oh, if you could find a nicer doctor, I would be so grateful!"

"And what about Aunt Nance?"

"She drove me to the doctor where I got the news. Then she drove me home. Then she had this stroke, right after."

Well, that makes sense. If we choose the time of our exit, as Bernie Siegel and others assert, so must we choose the time of many of our illnesses and accidents. Looking at my own life and the lives of my clients and students, it has certainly seemed so. Why should an eighty-year-old *not* have a stroke upon learning that her neighbor and niece is going to be needing a caregiver twenty-four hours a day? At least that's how it appears to me. My favorite aunt, a lifelong source of radiance and vitality, will not be available to me. She and my sister have always been major pillars for me. Now both are knocked out. I can feel myself teetering. I move slowly in a cloud of overwhelming anxiety.

"I will start searching right now and let you know what I find."

"They said I have to drink barium. I'll be terribly allergic to it. And to fast all day. I can't. I'm too weak. I haven't been able to eat solids in over a week."

"Stop fasting. Just take care of yourself. Rest. You won't have to go back to them. I'll find you someone here."

"Oh thank God. Thank you so much."

## July 29th

My vigil begins. I don't want radio or TV. I don't want to go out. I don't want to see friends, do anything, go anywhere. A compulsion to ready the house sweeps over me.

I have felt a need to come back to this historic house of my grandparents' for years. I would have, many times, but family schooling and career needs always loomed up as obstacles. We summered here many times. The boys went to camp next door. I turned most of the building into a counseling service to help pay the bills, while carrying out my mission at the same time and seeing this as a place where people could be taken care of.

Just feeling it the right time, I put our small, school-oriented house on the market (the best high school in the region just behind the woods in back) and sold it in one day, a day a colored kite landed in a tree outside my window and stayed. It was a time marked by synchronicities[2] (those luminous, unexplained coincidences on one's spiritual journey). The red plastic key holder holding the house-key for the past decade fell apart in my hands, a deer pressed its nose against the window like a friend watching me pack, strange signs all clustering together and feeling so right. This was the moment, and it all fell into place, lusciously.

One layer of my love for this house is historic—my own history in every corner and step. And a second layer—that it is a 1790 National Historic Site. Many families have lived here in rich, layered, chapters. But I also always knew it would be the ideal place to take care of people needing help and suspected my sister would be coming here in the end. I thought in terms of twenty years or so. I clean and scrub, feeling certain she is coming, now, although neither of us have said a word.

A part of me longs for a moment in which I will find it all a bad dream. Dee was quasi-ill all her life, the 'sickly one.' Please let it be exaggeration. But I don't think so, not this time. It was her quoting of the experts, both doctors, that both she and I knew would drive it home to me. I scrub the bathrooms, the huge kitchen floor, the pine scent giving me a feeling of satisfaction. Next I drag out the vacuum cleaner. Routine cleaning? Not at all. This is a ritual of some primitive kind. I can't put a name to it at all.

Ritual creation has become a specialty. Ancient cultures knew about rituals instinctively. Somewhere along the way of our Western scientific growth spurt we threw this wisdom out. Prayer, prayer baskets, throwing things out, visualization of a desired outcome. Even the Navy Eagle stunt fliers and Olympic ice skaters do it. All are being revived now simply because they work!

Not catharsis, preparation and prayer all in one. Nurses must feel this as they go about their day.

To rest, I place calls to friends who have had cancer for the advice only they can give. They jump to offer helpful suggestions;

Here's the number for my biochemist ... the guy who does guided imagery ... my surgeon's number.

They know the absolute terror. The hours of waiting with no

feedback. The desperation to know more. We are a silent club that no one wants to join, yet once in, appreciate so much.

Periodically, I call her. It has to be the worst day of her life. My sister, Dee, *can* this be real?

"That doctor was <u>so</u> nasty. I can not deal with him no matter what happens."

"Try not to worry. I'll stay on this all weekend. I'm going to find you a doctor you like." I know that the terror may be as bad as any physical parts.

"Oh thank you. So much."

"I'll let you know how I make out."

My friend Helen has just been through a year's ordeal. Her cat found her cancer in the course of a routine snuggle. The lump in the breast attracted her in some psychic way. Reiki and other esoteric body therapists claim that animals use their sharply-honed intuition to find disease. Now, Helen uses her cat as part of her healing environment. Patting and holding a pet raises the immune response and certainly manifests love and loving. She tells me now about her nutritionist, her body therapist. I take everything down carefully on a long legal pad that is filling rapidly with my scribbles.

My cat certainly knew what was going on in our household—both in our emotions and also when a family member would be starting home from some distant location. Our beloved Kato was an intuitive weathervane, we all came to know it.

Alan has five year's recovery from prostate cancer and has now been informed he has leukemia. "In remission," but still a neon sign to have over one's head. He gives me his surgeon's name and number. I consider how people's personalities are reflected in their response to a diagnosis. Some curl up and die. Others call out the troops. Others enlist a significant other and rely on them.

The sun sets, a golden glow over the Revolutionary burying ground behind my garden, silhouetting the darkened branches of trees against it. I feel the oldness in this place. How many souls have dealt with the exact same pains and fears, surprises and joys, right here, over the past two hundred years?

Some of the professionals, of course, never call back. I expected that. I call again and again. Finally, feeling a shade of desperation, I take answering service operators into my confidence. How that helps! I get some shoulders to cry on, and most of the messages do get answered after I've done it.

## July 30th

By late Sunday night, the last surgeon, an old friend of mine, calls back. It's very late and I know he's calling after a family weekend and that it's not fair to disrupt him, but that's what makes for a healing relationship—the old-time availability that patients used to be able to count on. I am so grateful I could cry. He describes possible surgery, but is just going on vacation. I ask about chemo and radiation for advanced colon cancer.

"Yes, chemo. A very low level dose is used several weeks after surgery. We could do it."

"What about a liver transplant?" I am really grasping at straws because I must save her. My brain is straining at every possibility.

"I'm afraid not, Cynthia, they save the few livers they can get for the young and healthy. She is not a candidate. Radiation also not helpful for her."

In spite of the horrible news, maybe, hope. It's so good to hear a familiar voice that it has undone me. But he can't do the surgery now because he'll be out of town, and it must be immediate.

So I'll keep looking. Now I reorganize myself, switching back into the therapist part of me and returning calls from my own answering service.

Responding to other people seems to give me renewed strength, so that I can think again.

Around eleven, a kind person calls from T.P.'s office. I've called there because I know she trained with Bernie Siegel. T.P. is away but he introduces himself and says, "The on-call person says I'm the sort you're looking for." Bernie has become a kind of password for a surgeon who will talk about love and hope and mix hugs and prayer with surgery. Thank God.

At present, much work is being done in the fields of psychoneuroimmunology and pain management. The first explores what lowers the immune response, which predisposes us to certain diseases like cancer. The second, how we can be less overwhelmed by pain. Everything from allergies to the severest pain can be made somewhat better or worse by emotions and tension. There is now a vast literature on this in book stores and online.[11]

One more call to bring Dee up to date. Let her know I'm on the job.

"He was so nasty, I can't go back to him."

She's repeating herself, poor thing. Panic does make the thoughts whirl round.

"I'll be out first thing tomorrow morning."

## July 31st

I drive out to Dee's house and she is not ready. Instead, she is chatting with a neighbor and seems to have all the time in the world. My stomach turns over with resentment. Responding to our emergency to rush to her aid, I have canceled an entire day of clients and my whole life. Yet, she chats on and says cheerily that she did not expect me so soon.

I sit in the car watching her, reflecting on the separateness of our lives. She's a little woman, with an Irish complexion and lovely blue eyes. From the looks of her, you would never guess she is sick. Pulling down her garage door at the same time as she hands a box over to her friend, she seems to be moving just as she always moved: quickly, tensely, efficiently, like someone who has been entirely on her own since Mother's death fourteen years ago.

We are both independent women with our own environments, activities and associates. We live over an hour apart. When I visit her, it is social, not intimate. And yet when I need help, she is always there. Gratitude, yes, she is always there. But she also infuriates, always stubborn, doing things her way, never willing to bend for another unless in the midst of their crisis. Then she's the one that gets the breakfast tray or the oxygen.

Now comes my first experience obliterating anger. There is no place for it whatsoever right now. Each time I feel it, I set it aside deliberately. It is a privilege somehow, deep in my heart, to be able to reciprocate in her crisis, no matter what.

At last, she is ready, calling out more things that her neighbor, Kaye, can do 'if she would,' and putting vitamins, basins, folders of papers, clothes, into my car. I see clearly that she is leaving her house for good. She hated this house and wanted to be out of there. We've talked about this for two years now. Her belongings are all shipshape, packed up, stashed in corners for a mover to come someday. Dee had spent her savings repairing this house, after finding that the seller had not been honest.

Buying it and losing so much money seemed to her a huge mistake. She longed to move South and be able to have us visit with children and grandchildren. And the merciless weather of the northwest comer of the state had finally gotten to her. It occurs to me this dreadful weight could have lowered her immune response and allowed a cancer to take root somehow. The potted plants on the porch seem to wave goodbye. I feel a giant lump in my throat. We start the hour-and-a-half drive to the hospital and chat.

"Remember when Mother took us for the ice cream soda and started laughing so hard she couldn't stop?"

"And the time Billy came over and he pronounced aunt (ant) as auwnt, and we both became hysterical?"

We've always traded jokes and cartoons. She has the wit of the Irish, and I have been trying to learn it. Our father's Irish heritage was a saving grace among lots of pathos. I admire her humor and have always sought its warmth.

We also talk about remedies, discomfort, allergies, and symptoms.

"Maybe your doctor is wrong. They can be, you know."

"I don't think so. But thank you so much for finding me someone kind. I could *never* go back to that other one."

This is the longest talk we have had alone since 1982. We are in a kind of time warp, picking up her crises, my crises, and a whole lot of stuff from our shared childhoods. I feel as though I am in a film.

She and I have been through so many crises since our very beginning, and she has so often erupted in anger toward many in the family that we have all become wary of her. But all of that is history, and this is right now. It is warm and protective inside this warp. Besides, being in the right hands make a universe of difference when one is terrified. She is obviously comfortable about that. I am so glad that I have the determination, and resources, to do this. We are going to the best hospital in the area. It is miles farther from her home and mine than others, but this is a time for the absolute best we can get for Dee.

We enter the ER at around ten a.m. The day of waiting begins. Here, they have a system where you may visit for ten minutes each hour. So I have a ritual that will mark the passing of hours, visiting her inside the labyrinthine emergency areas. Make calls, read, walk to the cafeteria, pass the time. Now I start to pray. I always pray when people are in desperate moments, and now I've learned that there are actually workshops on this. Knowing that there is research showing prayer's effects helps me enormously in the aloneness of the waiting room.[4]

The benches are arranged so that everyone seems to be isolated, and I hate it. The camaraderie I have found among folks in other emergency rooms and intensive cares is architecturally impossible in this one, which is set up more like a train. This architect has a lot to learn about life.

Three o'clock. I am starting to tire. If I were in the office, I'd meditate. Here I can only put my head back on vinyl and sigh. They announce my name—I startle. Inside, I look at Dee's pale face. How small she is! The news is that test results have arrived. I notice they are not sharing them with the patient. This can't be good. This hospital will redo the testing just to be sure. That's why we came here.

Dee's little white shoes poke up from out of the sheet: she seems to be shrinking. Mother dressed us alike when we were little girls in handmade smocked dresses of the same color, and everyone would look and exclaim, "how adorable!" But when we grew older, I wanted to look, and be, entirely different. She was "the sickly one," with special needs; and I was the one who "could do anything." Trauma would roll off me like water off a duck's back. I wanted my own dresses; and wearing them, I would go out in the world and do anything, rather than be part of a reclusive, troubled family. And so we moved into our own roles, and embellished upon them for years, becoming more and more the way we *thought* we were. Now, looking down at her, I feel a similar desire to reconnect to my own health, life and strength. In a word, to run away into my own personas. Yet how absurd, because three years ago I was the one in the hospital and she was my support. How strangely the mind bends and twists in its pathetic attempts to conquer a situation!

Many hours later, Dr. M. comes out to me. "So far, we've found no reason this should shorten life expectancy. Colon cancer is very common, and it is generally curable. We'll put her in the first bed that becomes available. But those tests, the cat scan, will be really critical. We'll schedule it as fast as we can, but she'll have to have that barium. I know how horrible this business can be. I've been through this in my own family." He put a hand on my shoulder, and I know I've found the right guy.

I go back in and say good night to the figure lying passively on the gurney inside. Although we've lived separately most of our lives, I feel so badly leaving her tonight. The nurse tells me I really should go.

It may be many hours before she is moved upstairs. I have no idea what to do, and am grateful for the advice. I kiss her as I would kiss a child.

Driving home in the dark, I realize that my car is full to the ceiling with her things, and that there is a strong medicinal smell I hadn't noticed. This is very, very, real.

## August 1st

I get a frantic call on my machine. "They've done a lot of tests. I'm scared. I need to hear from you."

She's afraid I've abandoned her. I can feel it in my bones. It takes five separate, agonizing calls to locate her in the giant medical center. I cannot get a nurse.

When I visit, she is white. "They insist I have to take the barium, but they say they'll monitor my allergies throughout. I'm still terrified of the citric acid I know is in it, but they say someone will be monitoring me the whole time. So I guess that's better. Did you bring me *anything* at all? "

She's testing me. Am I *really* going to be here? She lived with Mother for all but two years of her life. So she could always reach out and someone would respond instantly. And if she was in a panic, she could say something like that, 'did you bring *anything at all*,' and be sure to get a response. That was the nature of their relationship.

Now the legacy is handed to me, and I am scared. But I will not react to barbs. She can't believe that my steadfast presence is real. I know how it is. But I will prove myself! I bring—and will always bring her things. Things that will carry love and caring in their tangibleness. Today, it's the curlers and shampoo and address book. She is extremely grateful. Her possessions connect her to her life and herself. Dee's been in total control of her life until now, and it is hard to let go of all but one tiny strand. She tells me she'll be discharged five days after surgery. She's looking forward to coming to the old house with me. I feel a wave of nervousness.

## August 2nd

John has decided to both sand and paint the two rooms we are preparing for her. We buy a sander and paint, and he works for hours into the night. The strong cat smells from a previous caretaker's stay (and which resisted hundreds of dollars of professional cleaning) are completely gone! I rush out on a lunch hour and buy a bed that, they tell me, can be delivered in an amazing forty-eight hours! Now there's a cozy little suite complete with bath all ready in less than three days. So I tell myself we are doing all right! The anxiety about the stench, the lack of a bed, the whole task of room preparation, falls from me like a ton of boulders.

## August 3rd

They will operate tomorrow. Instead of becoming fearful, Dee is now very calm. Most of her energy goes into becoming fast friends with nurses, orderlies, residents, interns, as well as patients and their families. Can this be happening; that my shy, reclusive sister has changed to such an extent overnight? After a life alone, she has become the personification of loving community. The transformation is first startling, and then just beautiful. Watching her affectionate conversations with everyone she encounters, I feel sudden joy in the midst of my pain. Dee introduces me to her anesthesiologist, the med students, the girl across from her suffering a miscarriage, her husband, her mother.

I head home feeling a tangle of emotions. I am relieved that the operation is imminent. I feel as though I've been holding my breath over her starvation. She hasn't eaten solid food in over a week. After surgery, gradually, she will be allowed to eat!

All night I have nightmares about operations, body parts, running to help her, to help my children, my grandchildren, catastrophes and rescues. The torments in my dreaming are apparently what allows me to sleep, because I do.

**August 4th**

A telephone call from the doctor. He tells me they "did not remove the tumor. No point—it's all through her." So now he, too, has the hard truth. His former hopefulness obliterated. The heaviness of the news seems to squash me. I am uncomfortable about what he will say to her, but he seems the perfect soul for the task. Gentle. Soft spoken.

I am sitting next to Dee in her hospital room. When I had surgery, I had a private room. She is in a four-person one. I feel guilt over this dreadful, parsimonious insurance of hers. It was the reason she avoided doctors' offices. Visits weren't covered. If only she had said something!

But I've been in the hospital four times, and she has never visited me once. Topics jumble in my mind. Thoughts have catapulted from her meager insurance to my long-term feeling of having been abandoned by her. I'm getting used to my brain playing hopscotch and just try to stay centered and follow along. The four-person room is allowing her visible transformation; alone she could not become this loving communal presence her previous life never permitted. The Lord works in very strange ways! And as for her inability to ever visit me, "O.K., you had so many other people visiting it didn't matter." I coax myself—oh, yeah? I resolve to try let go of all differences and comparisons. They are only in the way of what we both need now: loving connection.

We talk over the surgery. She is in pain but has the shiny white patient-controlled pain medication dispenser at her fingertips and can use it as she needs. The anesthesiologist is "so sweet." He shows up again. He is from India and has a voice of honey. He holds her hand while he asks questions. I am secretly relieved when Dr. M. doesn't arrive during visiting hours: what will he say to her? All night, more bizarre dreams about Dee, blood, operations, but I'm so grateful for the sleep.

## August 5<sup>th</sup>

She does not tell me exactly what he has said, only, "It's all through me, there's no hope."

I tell her there is *always* hope—I'll send for the 'Spontaneous Remissions' literature from the Noetic Society. She has called Veronica for the Kushi diet things. Optimistic people who've been collecting all this stuff all our lives, we grasp at every straw of hope and promise. But there's a quiet about her that says, "very little chance of any miracles here." I try to support her mood of calm acceptance. She's coming to stay with me. This is the only way she wants it. A friend suggests 'Hospice Home Care services' in her own house and she says 'absolutely not.' There was something in the way she pulled down the garage door, with absolute finality, that signaled this to me. It's also payback time. She nursed Mother through an agonizing death, and she's also nurtured me all my life in many ways. (So long as I would come to her, by phone or in person—she wouldn't, couldn't, come to me.) Something inside me warms, is triumphant to have the capacity to give it all back now.

She gives me her watch. "The nurse says no jewelry in the hospital."

I wear her watch. Dee asks me to call her neighbor to be sure the lawn mowing man is paid in cash. Where does she leave off and I begin? Our identities are weaving together, as with a newborn baby, a child, a mother.

## August 6<sup>th</sup>

After work, John and I both come round with cars and pick her up with all the flowers, bags, clothes and gifts that have accumulated during the one week she's been in the hospital. On the way into the hospital, I am appalled when I see the patients attached to IVs, who have traveled all the way downstairs in their pajamas to smoke! Isn't life worth stopping for? Dee would certainly think so!

We are a sad little convoy pulling into the driveway next to the huge white Homestead, a few lights glowing from faraway windows, as we help her out of the car. When we first come into the house, I am very tense. My sister, who is three years older than I, always took charge quietly but firmly. We climb the creaky stairs slowly; she is extremely weak from surgery and not eating for so long even before it. She now takes the obligatory short walk into my room she's been told will help her regain strength and circulation and right away sniffs, "moth balls, carcinogenic," and gathers up four or five of my recovery-type books to take back to her room.

I rush to remove the offending clothes bags, running them down to the little storage room off the kitchen. (Where once grandmother housed a War Bride's entire family after the Second World War. Every inch of the house was used to care for someone. Now it's piled to the rafters with my move. Boxes I try to dispense with when I get time, my parents' and grandparents' estates, grown children's things from their rooms in our former home, years of career, historic papers. Another role I play: family legacy and archivist. This was to be the month for all of this: never mind.) I hardly notice that I am winded now from running up and down stairs to get her things, a blanket, a glass of water.

I breathlessly ask her what she would like for supper.

"I think I'll just try ginger ale and soup."

I notice that I am rounding up personal letters, journals, other private matters, fearing her intrusion into my intimate world. Since I was sent away to boarding school at thirteen, we've lived totally separate lives by choice—two Yankees from just such a family—and this trait has always been compounded in me by her criticalness. I've learned it can surface at any moment about food, safety, mothballs, appliances, my children. But enough of that! Something deep inside of me is struggling to adapt as quickly as possible, and one way may be trying to establish some privacy.

The tray is carried up with the only "dinner" she feels she can handle, and she retires, not to the new bed bought just for her and freshly made up with clean sheets, but rather to the couch along the end of the room. I notice but say nothing. It is only the first of the many little frustrations of trying to control an illness, or a person. I know this. The irony of my professional life—counseling, working with patients with life-threatening illness, teaching people to help others with "conscious dying"—is not lost on me. I can turn all this into a gift for Dee and I can learn from life what I need to learn.

Gradually, I must ease into this situation, let go of being in charge of every hour, every event.

"I am coming back to end where I began," she says with satisfaction.

I nod. "Yes. It's so right, isn't it. I'm glad I'm here and can do this."

"Thank you so much." This she will say every day for the remainder of her life.

"You're completely welcome. I know you'd do the same for me."

"I would."

"Do you still have the Grandfather clock?"

"I do. And it chimes, for the first time in twenty-five years! A client must have brushed against it one day and it crashed into a thousand pieces. When the clock repairman fixed the casing, I also had him do the works. Every time it chimes, I feel Grandfather's presence. It's lovely."

"Oh it must be!"

She is happy now, like a child opening a package and the package is this house, and me, after such a long time.

## August 7th

Very early, Adam, my youngest, calls from overseas. He has decided to get married in October. I know he has been longing for a loving relationship and marriage for some time, but the news is hard to absorb. I've heard about his new girlfriend, even talked with her. Now he goes on about his wonderful bride-to-be, how intelligent and caring she is. He is set on it. I am excited and enthusiastic, but through a pea-soup, unyielding, cerebral fog. I ask if he could postpone a bit under the circumstances. He doesn't think so, as he must go right into the army ten days after the ceremony. He apologizes for what this may mean for me and expresses concern over what Dee and I are going through.

Most of me is glad to get up, offer breakfast, go downstairs to the big 18th-century kitchen, mix up the cereal and make a big pot of coffee. It is pure joy to make food in this kitchen among spirits of grandparents, great-grandparents. I look out the window and into the historic burying ground where there are graves of townspeople from the 1600s. The white stones catch the sun. Making oatmeal is cozy, settling. Smells from childhood. Warmth.

This looking forward to August for such a long time, as the month when I would settle in here, this place I have longed to come back to for so long. Was this an intuitive precognition. Did I see, or feel, what lay ahead? There have been so many of these in life. Or was it just an incredible, ironic, coincidence? I will choose the first, it feels so true to me now. Synchronicities have paved the way of my life for many years now; I trust all my right-brain signals and hunches and use them, as my clients learn to, finding direction.

I'm extremely concerned about the food situation. When she was a baby, Dee was "the frail one." She lived on eggnogs to strengthen her tiny frame. I recently heard an expert talking about "sensitive babies" and how they must have "special handling" and a lot of support for years in order to "thrive." She never thrived. She must have been such a one, so frail and fearful, finding herself in a family where alcoholism and abuse settled in quickly, and she was scared out of her wits. She did *not* get that "special" handling of those experts, only spurts of over-protectiveness, interrupted by horror.

If only parents had known in those days how much help there

is in the outside world, but then again, dysfunctional households have precious little to do with that world—or even the world next door. (We never met our neighbors in the apartment building in New York. The only one any of us saw was the Jewish lady who screamed at night that the Nazis were coming to get her and escaped from her husband to run up and down the halls in her white nightgown—an appalling apparition for us. That was the world of the time in 3-D:[5] the Depression, the War and the Holocaust—and dysfunction!)

Dee tries calmly to explain to me all the things she doesn't eat. A little sigh escapes me.

"Citric acid, citrus, garlic, onions, chocolate," and then she protests, "but I really eat everything!"

Independent hardly says it. We come from a long line of fiercely independent immigrants. One set came on the Mayflower, the other left Ireland's poverty. When our father died, Mother was impoverished. She rented out half the refrigerator, and her bedroom, to a complete stranger. I have no words for how that feels when you are thirteen and no one tells you what is happening until you walk right into that wall. We were astonished and afraid. No relatives came forward to help Mother. This, unfortunately, was the Puritan way. Our Anglo-Saxon forebears had left everyone behind when emigrating. After arriving in the New World, they also threw off British rule and the Anglican religion. Some of the first "radical" new colonial churches are within a block of this house! Can it be that we descendants of early Americans have a genetic disposition toward family dispersion? We certainly keep a "stiff upper lip" and expect folks to make it on their own, like the early settlers! This can make everything harder at a time like this.

Marty, the visiting nurse, came today. Such a comfortable woman, I feel as though a best friend has dropped by. She brings literature on the agency, folders, cards, handouts. But I neither see nor hear any of the details. When I tell her of my panic looking ahead to the wedding in October, she says, " This is August. That's October. Don't worry now. That's a long way away."

I lean against the pantry door, the area where we can escape to talk. These are precious moments for me, a new and predictable time for support. I can read between these lines. She's saying it may well be over by then. I feel a visceral shudder.

## August 8th

I wake up early and ask Dee what she wants for breakfast. I have started asking prior to each meal, if you can call three bites a meal, because everything I take up goes back down to the kitchen. The hope of her eating after surgery has faded for us both. No one told us, obviously because those last strands of hope are so precious. A small chunk of bread, a cup of coffee, a bowl of soup. If she manages a bite, or a swallow, it's a triumph.

"I'd like to try some oat bran with chopped dates. And just a sip of coffee."

I trot down to the kitchen and make the cereal and coffee and bring it up.

"Oh dear, you've used the *wheat* bran." Her twenty unmarked jars of health food and the two dozen vitamins brought from her house confuse me completely. A 'Health Person' can drive you crazy. But now, the rules have changed completely. Her liver is gone.

Yesterday, she got excited about coffee and vanilla ice cream. I rushed out for supplies. She had it twice. The third serving "didn't work." She could not get it down. I notice today it's "just a sip" she's asking. I've asked her what this is like. "Like the flu, only twenty times worse."

"I'm sorry. I'll try again." Now I descend once again and make the other "correctly" this time. The Little Sister in me always trembled at doing things wrong. It is a subpersonality[10] I am very familiar with!

She sees the pain on my face. "I have these nice little plastic baskets. If you use them, you can save lots of steps."

It's a great idea. I feel better. Big Sister helping.

Only once did my sister come to visit. It was when I was a beginning housewife with small children, She threw out all of my clutter, much of my food and a number of things I cherished—and we both became very upset. Afterwards, she and I tacitly decided to leave it at that. Not only did she never visit me again, she didn't visit any relative until Aunt Nance became old and infirm, and then it was to be helpful, a role in which she excels. Instead, we traveled to *her* house, where she was the perfect hostess, with home-made baked goods, a beautifully set table and lots of surprising little details, like her own plant seedlings as gifts for us to take home.

The nervousness is still with me when she walks into my room on her "circulation walks." I continue to gather up journals, letters, and papers, putting them in storage, haunted by times many years back, when other relatives have lain dying, and she has thrown out and given away their things mindlessly. "Why doesn't anyone tell you that when you run a Home Hospice all the ghosts of family history will rise to the surface like corpses in a lake? Or that, when someone you love has cancer in their liver, the twenty trips to the store will be fruitless, and how nothing, yes, nothing you do will make any difference except at the level of love? A wave of desperation. I quiet it.

Tonight, I confess I ate cold potatoes in the bathroom, sitting on the edge of the bathtub. Why? Because I had the plate in my hand and was too exhausted to go anywhere else to eat. I was just too exhausted to make it back down, one more time, to the refrigerator or the stove.

## August 9th

Dee was the parent when I was little, and my parents unable to do the job much of the time. How many meals, freshly cooked, delivered on a tray? How many pieces of advice. "Better take vitamin C so you don't get that cold any worse," or "You have to slow down," or "He's no good for you," always delivered firmly, humbly, directly.

I remember her presence, like a watchdog, in our childhood

home, always hovering. When some of my friends drank too much at my New Year's Eve party, she was the one who declared the party over.

"If I could *just* get down to the kitchen to make myself a sandwich. I want to be a good patient for you."

"You are a fine patient," I protest, remembering those thousand trays carried to me in my room, or bed. "You were more mother than Mother." I say it, and once I also wrote it to her in a note so that if something happened to one of us, she would know my gratitude.

She thanked me when that note arrived. Just as she thanks me again, every night. She's never missed a night.

We trade memories when I come into her room. I sit by the window, she lies against the pillow in the bed.

"Remember the time they took us to that great film on Africa? "

"Vaguely, yes. It was so late at night and I was so tired. I remember falling asleep in all the reading aloud of bedtime stories too!"

"Well, you were three years younger. No wonder! That one was a classic film. They took us to lots of great ones, like *Bringing up Baby*.

"I'd completely forgotten that we went anywhere." There's lots I don't recall. They say that goes hand-in-hand with a lot of pain in one's early years.

"You are thinking of a time a few years later, when Poppy started to fall apart."

"I do remember Poppy bringing toys and candy when he came out on weekends, little dolls and gold-wrapped boxes of chocolates from Grand Central station. I've always wondered what it was like for those men in the forties and fifties, the weekend fathers. Don't you think it could have contributed to all the drinking and marital problems? Husbands were abandoned work horses! How tragic. Did he ever abuse you? I've always wondered about that. You were alone with him so much."

Dee replies without hesitation, "I never let him. I looked at him one day and decided, 'This is my parent in name only. I *can* have a decent life.' I used to fight him off with a chair held up so the legs pointed out at him. But you know about the time he strangled me, because you saved my life!" She looks out the window at some faraway thought, much farther away than the iron gates to the cemetery, or the street light back there that is glowing like a moon against the late afternoon sky.

We both sit in silence. I am back there now. First outside in the hall, Mother's weak hands restraining me, while I knew in my bones something was terribly wrong in the bedroom. Then, breaking my mother's innocent weak grip, as she was all obedience and could never go against her husband. With a karate move that Poppy himself had taught me, breaking free and smacking through the shut door, dashing into the bedroom and beating him off with my fists, while my sister lay helpless in the bed. I clearly saw his hands around her throat and the white and red fingerprint there, after. I shake, even now, remembering. Was that the day I met my will?

The depth of Dee's anger toward our father astonished me at first, as all these hurtful details have resurfaced (as they always will, when one spends sustained time with family). The hours tiptoe by, and I begin to understand in my body as well as my mind. I had at first expected her to be very attached to the father who chose her as "the one who truly understood" his private hell. For our father, Mother and I were "dizzy blondes" who would probably die of polio. (A death sentence to my ears, for no vaccine yet existed.) I found myself in awe of the phenomenon of her survival. So this is how a frail child made it through a childhood full of alcoholism, emotional neglect, marital discord, physical abuse, battered-wife syndrome, divorce, and her father's final death from an overdose of alcohol and barbiturates! We have professional terms for all this stuff today, criticized as jargon perhaps. But at least the skeletons are out of that stuffed closet! All those years, I carried the family burden of silence, like a heavy weight across my shoulders, always aching, no wonder.

Two members of the family came in the evening, and for the first time she left all the lights off. I felt absolutely shocked by this symbolic change. We all sat in the dark with her talking in subdued voices. The dark is closing in on us.

When each visitor leaves, I take them into the dining room where Marty has helped me discover I *can* talk freely. This is where we face emotions ready to burst. They ask how bad it is, and I tell them. We hug and we cry. Tonight, it is my ex-husband. He has come a long distance to say his goodbyes. We stand and talk, not realizing one of our sons has sneaked back up for a longer goodbye and private hug with Dee. His father says now, "Well, about the wedding invitations. Does it matter that they're in a foreign language?"

"Not at all," I answer, thoughtlessly, realizing that there are no older family left for me.

"... and Aunt Nance is aphasic now, so what's the difference," interrupting my thoughts. His parents are also long gone. We both start to giggle unexpectedly. My giggles mix with tears before I even know this is happening—emotional Jell-O mix.

## August 10th

She tried so hard to eat today, diluting strawberries in seltzer. I note that she has begun to dilute even her *soda* with water. She pours the liquids back and forth with great concentration. They are her connection to life. How ironic this is. A woman who started cooking as soon as she could reach the stove, who was The Chef for the family, passionate about food and creating recipes, has lost a favorite dimension to living. She had few others. She is a frail, little figure, sitting huddled up in the couch in the dark tonight.

## August 11th

"I abandoned you when you were two and Great-Grandmother died. I was supposed to stay here with you. You stood under the apple tree and just wailed." Dee says these things out of the blue, very much like my five-year-old granddaughter. They are angels, innocent, honest, open.

I recall this as though it were last Tuesday. They'd left me with an unknown person, a huge cook in a white uniform. All I knew was that the whole family had left in a car. It was total abandonment and forever to me then. But there was another, much worse, in 1948, when my family left me and did *not* return. My sister made the phone call. She simply said, "We're leaving."

Mother and Dee then went to Reno for the obligatory six months on a ranch. While I knew it was required by law for a divorce, "ranch" sounded like fun. Postcards would arrive talking about the great new friends made out there. I felt as though everyone had left the planet.

I stood in a small telephone booth in the night at a Vermont boarding school and cried my eyes out. It was not really a surprise that Dee had been the caller. She was the only one capable of any emotional availability. And I could hardly tell anyone at school, because no one was on that kind of intimate level there. It was a place where you felled a tree or lugged a garbage can. You didn't say much. I told my roommates, my best friend, my boyfriend, sobbed, buried it. From now on I would "dissociate" from pain, a trick hurt children are skilled in!

In the spring, I got some hope. Father wrote from his hospital bed. "Let's get together and start a new life." And the school said Mother would come to visit Sunday afternoon. I felt like dancing!

When that Sunday afternoon came around, Mother appeared mysteriously out of a taxi. We walked for a minute or two. Then she turned to me. "Poppy died in his sleep. You're coming with me to the funeral."

"Poppy." I always wondered where this unusual name came from. Then, at a seminar on alcoholism, a social worker delivered a heart-wrenching tribute to his alcoholic Irish, father, "Poppy." I wept and realized for the first time that this was another small piece in the mosaic of Irishness he never was able to share with his daughters.

Flowers at the florist with a card signed "Betty and the girls." Mother's gloves soaked through with the tears she could not cry? She didn't know what to do for me. She couldn't talk, or weep, so she took me to buy a dress. A special Valentine's dress for me with a curved neckline bordered with a velveteen ribbon ...

All day, Dee tries to think of things she can swallow, and all day I run to get them from the kitchen, where shelves and closets are beginning to overflow, or from stores five or ten miles away. Saving trips up and down the steps with plastic baskets was her idea for people who can wait, and now we can't. We both think her sudden impulses of foods, like a pregnant woman, *may* be things that can go down right now. So I'll dash out like the husband any hour of day or night. But no convenience stores where I live, and how I could use some "convenience"!

Lists of things for her neighbor to do, lists for me to do, lists of things to buy or get. Lists mark my days like lines on a sheet of paper. And there is no space left for me, the writer, to write of me.

"Ask Kay to do the dishes in the sink at my house. And please to leave a light on in the kitchen window. Pay the lawnmower man in cash."

Tonight, as every night, she sets her hair in little clips all over her head. She still has the will to do this. It is amazing.

## August 12th

Marty and I have worked out a nice schedule. She comes three times a week and brings her own special cheerfulness and objectivity. She is like an island in a bleak, cold sea. We always chat just off the kitchen on her way out.

"You don't need to *try* so hard. It's the liver. Appetite goes, no matter what. You don't think she would ever settle for Hospice?"

"I doubt it. She really wants to die here at home."

"Well, you take care of *yourself*. It's *hardest* on professionals."

"Why?"

"Because everybody assumes that you know, and can do, everything."

Like a broken necklace, bits and pieces of me have spilled and then disappeared. My music? My usual feelings and satisfactions? My passion for gardening? Now the flowers seem to call me, but there are only tiny slices of moments. I say goodnight to them when I water the garden. It brings me down to earth and soothes me. It is like holding my Self for just a moment before dark sets in.

In addition to my own calls, all Dee's friends and neighbors now telephone me. The phone seems to ring non-stop. She gives me tasks off a neatly written page on a yellow pad. I need to talk to her real estate agent about her house, and to a kindly neighbor about a tag sale. She also asks me to call the lawyer and the accountant. I don't know if I can manage all this. I feel overwhelmed.

Each time someone calls for her, I lean back in my chair, look up and summon all of my spiritual resources. I learn something new: how much the callers can help. One says, "She always brought us cookies." Another, "We looked forward to her visits so!"

I think of *Jack*, a movie that John and I saw last week while Dee was in the hospital. She doesn't like it when I go out now. A condition of time-acceleration has propelled this character into old age, while his school classmates are still in high school. Someone comments that "Some souls are just so special, they are like shooting stars—here for a short while but making such a blaze across the sky." I weep all through this film. This is the way I think of my sister: a little star, sweeping across the sky, soon to be gone, and one that I and the world missed most of, because of her hiding out deep inside her home, and herself.

## August 13th

Dee is like a shadow. "I feel you let me down when Mother was sick, I feel you didn't come through," curled into the corner of the couch. It's time for unfinished business. She has a dark expression.

"I think you forgot because you were understandably upset and burned out."

I have to remind her of painful details, details I've buried for some time. "Do you remember my driving five hours to meet her at the nursing home so she'd feel more cared for when she arrived? Or visiting on weekends. It was close by for you, but over four hours for me. Yet, I *did* it. Or the day you said you 'couldn't handle it,' and I had to go to Danbury Hospital to meet her arriving on a stretcher and help her in telling the doctor she wanted no more treatment? That she was ready to start dying? You said you couldn't handle it. I couldn't either, but I *had* to. That was the worst moment of my life. I couldn't stop crying all the way home and for days after."

I speak slowly because it is hard to find the next breath. "And all the times I called the Hospice medical director about her care? He was wonderful. They never charged me, even though they couldn't take her in those days because of the oxygen tank. I've donated every year since. I think you forgot all the things I was doing because it was so horrible for you. You were on the firing line, so to speak, the caregiver, and, believe me, *I understand.*"

"Yes." A long pause. "That was good for us. Now I feel better. Don't you?"

"Yes, of course. It's important for us to clean up all that stuff and just get rid of it now."

I could go on and on with my unfinished business, like the time ... but I am hale and hearty and she is emaciated and exhausted. We are like musicians playing a duet that she must direct. She takes these things in micro doses, but they work for her. That's what counts. I may be a therapist with a bag of credentials, but no one ever told me that in the last stretch, little acts of reconciliation go such a long, long way.

## August 14th

Today she stood at the top of the stairs to say something, and what I saw was an ambulatory skeleton. It frightened me to see bones outlined in flesh. She has not eaten solid food in more than a month. I am using the little plastic baskets now when I can. It is now possible to insert thought into my succession of actions, and they save many trips up and down the stairs. Also, they are from my Big Sister, and that means a lot symbolically. She's always been there in times of spiritual crisis, and this is one, and she still worries about me and cares for me like the Little Sister that I am. Occasionally, she will say, "Can you get some *rest* now?" I have finally gotten enough wits about me to have her make a list of things she can't eat:

> citrus
> citric acid
> tomatoes
> oranges
> grapefruit
> onions
> garlic
> chocolate
> monosodium glutamate
> aspirin
> kiwis
> sulfa
> penicillin
> cheddar cheese

A critical part of me wonders if she really is allergic. In the hospital they insisted she take citric acid in the barium, and she was fine. They also gave her suspicious-looking juices and sodas without the labels. Oh well, who cares. I turn that off like a switch and prepare to make my daily trip to the stores. It is possible to turn it off; you just have to want to badly enough.

When I return, she always tries whatever it is, and always with renewed hope. I bring her root beer, gherkins, like offerings to a queen. We have supper. The tray will have two bites taken, the rest goes back untouched. Now that I know in advance, it is less terrifying for me. I wonder how it is for her.

"I tried," she looks up at me, child-like.

"I know you did," I answer, lovingly. "Just do what you can. We'll see."

This is a soul who, although very close to poverty, checked "Operation Fuel" every month on her utility bill so that a poor family would have some help. Every month.

## August 15th

Dee has started talking about "taste." <u>Very</u> specific ideas. Could I just run out and get some Progresso minestrone? And, "I'd like to try ginger snaps. Taste. Anything with taste. I *love* to eat, but not now."

It breaks my heart to see her try so hard. As an anorexic child, she laid down a ground of self-consciousness about not eating. Now she struggles against it. C.S. Lewis speaks of anger at God over hope. I have a different view. Hope creates more of those good, comfortable, cheerful moments, and aren't they all that any one of us can be sure of? In some, they also raise the immune response, but we both know we're too late for that now.

Even sweet Marty is not impervious. She brings a large clump of parsley for "the taste." It's from her own garden. One has to believe that life lies within the moments, not the endings.

## August 16th

Dee's ready two hours early for the doctor's appointment. She and Mother, both cursed with an overload of anxiety, conscientious to a painful extreme, wore their lives like leather gloves, with little room to move about in at all. They both admiringly described me at times as the "taxi driver," able to manage any expedition, any traffic, any parking. So, of course, I seldom told them about my own anxieties, moments of trauma. When you wear the role of "intrepid" in a family, it's very hard to step outside it.

Driving around the block five times to find this "very convenient" office, we get exasperated. We can't find a sign, or any attendant in a parking lot, or office building doorway, who could get us a wheelchair. We finally spot an entrance from the wrong side of the street and, since we're late, she volunteers to walk it, weak as she is. My heart pounds with anxiety. Dee gets out and walks across the street. A thousand memories follow her like autumn leaves. It is the last time I will see her walk, in street clothes like an ordinary person.

When I park the car and locate her, she's white as a sheet and has collapsed into a wheelchair inside the doorway. I, wrapped in my cheery, confident manner, push the wheelchair, aware of a crowd pressing behind us, and bump into things, doors, ramps, the side of the elevator. It feels like a thousand yean since I worked in a medical setting where wheelchairs were familiar. It is huge, completely unwieldy, and she's a tiny little sparrow inside it.

"Careful!" she admonishes me. I an embarrassed, five years old, totally back in my Inner Child trying to care for Big Sister and not knowing quite how to do it. Thank God, I've learned all about subpersonalities, how to tap their wisdom and step outside of the vulnerabilities of each.

In the doctor's office, everyone stares. I know what they are thinking, it must be really bad if they need a wheelchair. I have to bring her all the forms and questions. Then take them back to the little window where the clerk sits. All forms of support are hidden behind glass and cubicles. This is an odd feeling. I have become her legs and strength. One becomes attached by a psychic umbilical cord. Always two. We breathe together, move together, our existences braided together like little girls' hair.

Finally, we are taken into the inner sanctum. The kindly doctor invites me into the cubicle. Dee asks me not to look at the surgical scar.

"I promise I won't."

I put my head down during the physical examination. My promises are made of steel these days. Nothing can stop them as long as I am alive.

"Thank you," she says once again from above me, where doctor and nurse are examining surgical scars, removing sutures, making small talk about "Ensure" and other things she might be able to get down.

"My son thinks it's the greatest milkshake."

We emerge, and he says goodbye to each of us with a hand on the shoulder. To her, "You are doing fine. See you September 10th." There is not a moment's hesitation. When you are taking care of someone this sick, you find your senses are getting so acute you can pick up caring and trying on newly sensitive radar wherever you go. I wonder what he is thinking. This would be getting close to the end of our two months. Will we be back at all?

To me, a warm press on my right shoulder. "You are doing a wonderful job."

The words melt me like butter. I remember how he told me he's been through this in his own family. Was it his father? His wife? Brother? He really feels what it is for us both. I want to cry, but I can't. I wouldn't be able to see to drive.

On the way home, I'm hoping she'll go for McDonald's. She may never have been to one. But I only have two hours to get her fed, into bed at home, and myself back to the New Haven office to see a client at three. I am stretching my clients out as far as I can without hurting their process, but this one must be seen. Dee is enthusiastic, and I get two sandwiches for her, hoping one will be "all right." She samples both and likes the McChicken best. "It's delicious!" She is like a little girl. I am pleased with myself. It reminds me of the story in *Winnie The Pooh* about Tigger's breakfast.

Tigger had no idea what he liked, so he sampled each one of his friends' breakfasts in turn, but would then sadly shake his head and say, "No, that was not what Tiggers eat for breakfast." Finally, he went to the home of Kanga and Roo where Roo was eating breakfast and Kanga poured out a big spoonful of extract-of-malt which he must take because he was so tiny. Tigger tasted it, and his eyes lit up. At last, he'd found what Tiggers eat for breakfast! We both have a good laugh.

A memory: a party. We've all been invited and, incredibly, my parents have said we'll go. It is the only party we ever attended outside the immediate family. It's the Fourth of July, and I am so excited, a social butterfly even at this young age! Not ten minutes into the party, our cousin blows his finger off with a firecracker. Dee is halfway to the car in terror. Our parents scoop us up and back home. I am devastated. I wonder if she understands *me* at all.

## August 17th

Marty looks at me—dark circles under my eyes, chaos in the kitchen, laundry on the floor.

"You need help."

"Help!" I nearly collapse. "There's *help*?

"Oh yes, but your sister didn't want it."

"Why not?" I wonder if Dee is losing her mind.

"She said she likes it just the way it is."

I pour out my heart to Marty like a river overflowing its banks, about the twenty trips to the store, the laundry, the running of this nineteen-room-counseling-center- historic site. The garbage cans that have to be dragged out, the lawn, the shrubs, the clock that must be wound, plants watered, newspaper recycling, the cleaning service that won't do the residence area, the caretakers' breakdown and departure, the twelve counselors, the clients.

She gets it. "I know! I'll put it in terms of your needs. She'll never accept it on the basis of *hers*."

Marty worked her skills I'm sure and would have brought her around quickly. But tonight, Dee tried to wash her hair in the sink. When I came upstairs with the fifth snack she was attempting, I found her on the floor, towel wrapped round her head, eyes shut. For an endless moment, I thought her dead. So fast? So sudden? But we hadn't *finished!*

Then she spoke. "Don't be frightened. I just got very woozy. I shouldn't have washed my hair."

"Let's get you up very slowly and back to bed." I support her with hands under her arms and we make it.

"I can try the bed now. I only used the couch because my stitches seemed to bother me less curled up against it. Now there's no pain."

She never mentioned the pain at the time. I resented her not using the new bed that I had struggled to get in time and never realized how she was suffering. She is incredible! I take her in to the bed, tuck her in. Wish her a good night. Back in my own room, I marvel that she still has washed and set her hair daily. It is the human will, ever present, not giving up. She does a visualization she's created out of one of the books I use for training, *Getting Well Again*.[8] This technique is believed to have raised the immune response for some patients with tumors if the model is one they create and like. An animal lover all her life, Dee's made an assembly line of little animals on a carousel. Each one on the line carries away one cancer cell. She reads all of Bernie's books; they form a little pile at the end of the bed. And the Kushi Institute material is stacked there, too, although someone told her it was too complicated for her to bother to follow, so she never did.

I lie back against the pillow and try to imagine what is it like to have less than two months. After those very few days of anguish, protest and distress, she's moved to a different plane. We both hear the clock ticking, but our perceptions must be completely different.

**August 18th**

Marty says she will talk Dee into getting some help immediately. After last night, there is no longer any question.

Returning from work, I go in to see if she's agreed to having an aide at last, and she says, "I'm so sorry to disrupt your life this way."

"This is my life. I wouldn't have it any other way." I *mean* it.

She knows it.

Cousin Shirley will visit today. Just the thought of it makes us emotional. When we were girls, she was like a third sister, five years older than me, two years older than Dee. She lived with our grandparents here in the house and often was part of our family for weeks at a time. She has come to visit our aunt who is recuperating from the stroke at rehab. Shirley has crossed the entire continent just to lend her, and us, support. We all have tears in our voices as we try to cheerfully reminisce about the childhood days.

"Remember when you ate the worm between two slices of toast?"

"Yes, oh yes, and the time Granny drank the flower water from all the vases that the maid had just left out in the kitchen!"

The big hurricane when we drove to Granny's with trees crashing in front of us across the road ... singing harmony on the fallen tree in the woods ... the ice man bringing a huge boulder of ice to cram into the top of the wooden ice box ... camping out in the pup tent and giggling through the night.

Laughter feels so good. It also keeps us from getting more intense than we care to get. I dash out to do some errands. They have piled up into scary, teetering stacks in my imagination, as Dee is too anxious to let me leave without always a "how long do you have to be gone *this* time?" (A slight note of panic accompanied by another of accusation, "You are leaving me too much. Please don't, not even if they are essentials.")

I never had a child like this one. I wonder how Mother could deal with the tension and the guilt of it all. They lived together the major portion of their lives. This rattles me sufficiently that I make a call on the cell phone while I'm out to ask what I should get for lunch just to provide tangible proof to Dee that I am within reach every time I leave, using this marvelous new technology. She is amazed that it works, just as she was thrilled by being able to charge her calls to my charge card earlier. She is an old-fashioned country girl. The new world is scary and complex.

Dee says, very proudly, "Cinny has restored one piece of furniture every year," to all the guests.

I am delighted to see that she is now feeling a part of, and pleased with, all this.

"It looks great!" Shirley says, to support her cheeriness. She will sit with Dee while I get out to a meeting. I feel relief throughout my body unexpectedly. I hadn't realized I was so tense or exhausted.

My friend Marilyn drops by with an armful of flowers for Dee that are intense, celestial, blue, just like the blaze of her personal warmth, and with a dress she thinks one of us might enjoy. Her hug feels so good to me.

We travel to an open meditation meeting, something we do once a month to stay connected as a spiritual community during the summer months when there are no classes. Just being in the hostess's home, looking out at her beautiful trees, I listening to her melodious voice as she reads a meditation from Steven Levine[9], our breathing takes us to a place of calm and peace, letting go of our worries and fears and just being here.

I feel renewal seeping into me. I had no idea how burned out I had become already. It's been less than a month. The tension in me is like twisted rope. Releasing it from one area of my body at a time, I let in the sunshine, the love radiating in this meditation circle. I am so grateful. A tear slips down my cheek. This time I let it.

When we return, Shirley and Dee have had a satisfying visit. They have actually toured the entire house and garden. Not knowing her weakness, Shirley has cheered Dee all over the place, and Dee has risen to the occasion. Shirley is a grandmother who is still teaching a full day, getting up at five to swim each morning, and has never experienced anything to do with weakness or collapse, even when losing her husband suddenly in the midst of his cardiac surgery.

It is Sunday, so there are no clients or counselors, and, inspired, Dee has rallied incredibly. They are both enthusiastic about the things I've done. Neither has seen the place since 1968, when Granny left it to me, the youngest, because everyone else said "no" to the responsibility of this mansion and the weight of family and town history. I feel the appreciation like warmth on my skin, after years and years in this project.

Downstairs, I take Shirley into the dining room. We both start to cry. The house and all its furnishings put symbolic arms around us ... the captain's chair brought back from Canton in the China trade by Captain John, the faded oriental rugs we sat on as little girls to play with a delicate china doll who actually walked when wound up with a key (*poupee qui marche* from the Paris World's Fair). We are flooded with a confetti of memories as we hug goodbye.

"I'll be back," Shirley says, reassuringly, but who knows when.

## August 19th

Dee has taken in the entire environment in her one tour: Grandfather's books on the library shelves, the broken music box Uncle Charles brought back from Europe just before the Second World War, the bird bath I've had inscribed as a memorial to a number of relatives who have lived here. She's especially appreciative of the care manifested in these details, as she's thinking a lot about legacies.

I ask her if she has any special wish. "Just do something in the gardens with some of my money. That's what I'd like."

Sunday's rally was a great effort for her. Today, Dee is so tired she doesn't go for a walk. It is the same way with food. She was so pleased with a specific kind of soup she had me run out last night and get for her that she ate it all, and today we have a new problem. "I overdid. I ate too much. It's very uncomfortable. I must *never* do that again."

On the tour with Shirley, Dee spotted a hornet's nest on the back porch high up under the rafters. "You've *got to get* hornet spray, and I'd like to take care of it. We can't have the children getting stung."

Can this be? She wants to do it? She's too weak to sew curtains or to make a phone call, but *she* will do this?

"Be sure it's twenty-five-foot spray. Nothing less potent. And while you're out, I will also pay for a tub mat. We don't want poor little

Tory slipping in your tub." The children and grandchildren are coming for a "goodbye visit."

I am excited and touched, yet this control side of her is alienating. Today, I feel very uptight. I go to four stores before finding exactly what she wants. I am very, very tired. I wonder how long one can keep up the pace.

"Could you just bring me *one* glass of soda to mix with my water. Oh dear, I promised myself I wouldn't ask you for stuff when you've just climbed back up all those stairs. I'm sorry. I'm not going to do that again!"

"That's all right. I'll get it." But while I do, I am wondering if a schedule for the two of us would help, perhaps of meals, and snacks, and phone calls, so we could both get some sort of a rhythm going.

## August 20th

After three days unable to leave her bed from exhaustion from the walk, Dee says, "Tonight, we'll do the wasps. It has to be exactly at sundown or they won't be in the hive, and it's a waste of effort."

This is the biggest part of my sister. The Country Person who knows literally all there is to know about farms, nature, plants, vermin, and animals. And throw into the mix health remedies, cooking, nutrition.

I am incredulous, but when I drop by, very casually, to check at the appointed hour to see how she's doing, she's standing up and wearing her raincoat! We descend the stairs and venture out onto the porch. Here she takes the 25-foot spray can from my hand, stands on a table, and decimates the wasps. We both go back inside quickly so as not to inhale any "cancerous" vapors, as she insists, giggling over the irony.

"I think I'll also stop flossing my teeth. I mean, what for?" We are both convulsed with laughter. She follows me into the front room of the huge house, where I perform the ritual of winding our Grandfather's clock. As I move the little hands slowly, just as I was taught, she hears its chime for the first time since she's been here. It is an indescribable moment. As children, we stood a thousand times while Grandfather did this slowly, painstakingly. Today, we would call this mindfulness and teach it in a workshop to frazzled Americans. The experience is many centuries old, and Grandfather was a master of it in his own way, winding a clock, binding a book, searching out a star while standing in the darkness on the flat part of our spacious roof.

"Every time I do this, I feel as if he's inside the clock."

"I know," she nods so understandingly.

Objects entice her back into our shared past. On a Sunday night, one can wander in the rooms, even in a nightgown, and see the perfection reserved for the public all week long. We are like people in the Great Houses in England, I imagine, consigned to live in one small room, wrapped in their "woollies," who may not have a dime, but refuse to give up, so they put their houses to work. Well, some of the same blood is in our veins.

This is only the second time in all these weeks she has felt the strength to see the first floor ... drawers in desks that when opened release grandparents' smells of tobacco, must and perfume ... the urn in the drawing room brought back from China by Captain John ... the dining room table made in Barbados during the Depression for thirty dollars ... threadbare rugs, Orientals trod by generations of family and thousands of clients ... the highchair recently restored for my grandchildren, where, as babies, we both ate so many meals.

I over-water the many plants from the counseling service area while she chats with me. I apologize; "Oh look! I've over-watered as usual."

"Tell me about it. I always over-watered." Now, everything she says is in the past tense. It is a jarring note at first. "I was planning to make a quilt." "I would have liked to have invited the grandchildren to my house."

It stops me cold. And yet at the same time, we can chuckle over water trickling across oak flooring. Now we turn off all the lights, lock the door, and return back up the stairs, my hand under her shaking arm. I am so glad to have shared the fresh air of the outdoors, the wonders of the downstairs rooms so far from her own, the completeness of the restoration with her.

## August 21st

The Psychosynthesis Institute is giving a benefit, and the organizer has set up a phone radio interview. She will give all the particulars for time, place, fee, workshop descriptions and, since they all know my predicament, all I have to do is ramble on about transpersonal psychology and our specialty within this field.

I take care of Dee, get my granddaughter Tory settled with my dollhouse and check with my answering service. There's a message: "You have to do the interview on your own. Penny has a crisis and can't make it."

I race for the portable telephone, knocking the entire dish drainer into the sink, breaking a number of things, and dash upstairs to hide in my room where people can't ask me things during the interview if it *has* to happen. Thank heavens that Marty happens to be here. After ten minutes, the radio hostess has still not called. So I call her.

"Oh thank goodness. I lost your number!"

Breathlessly, I explain.

"Oh no. Can't possibly postpone. (She's as frantic as I am.) I'm booked every minute. We just *have* to do it now."

"I don't have the details. Penny was managing all that because I am running a Home Hospice. She told you?"

"We have to do it anyway."

And so it goes. I slip into some kind of altered state and ramble on. Before I know it, it's over. The words have simply passed through my lips, sent by an angel.

Rosio, the health aide, is another God-send. She is pleasant and soft. Ever since the incident where I found Dee on the floor, she has been assigned to us. After that, it did not have to be put in terms of my needs, although they seem monstrous to me. When she enters the house, I feel better immediately. Sometimes she's late, but I don't care. That she is coming at all and that it is free of charge to the dying feel like miracles.

Jet-black curly hair and a mellow voice. She is capable and very calm. I am delighted that her background is Hispanic, because I have a strong, synchronistic affiliation with that culture, and I find myself hoping to become great friends with her. To share a cup of coffee, to invite her to the retreats we run in the Spanish Virgin Islands, to learn Spanish with her, to really know her in a deep way. Dee worries that she'll "have to see my scars, but I guess she needs to be used to that for her career."

"That's right," I assure her. My sister is a very private person.

She has never wanted me to see those scars, and I've respected that. When you have surgery or cancer, you can say goodbye to modesty in general. But if she can hold onto one tiny piece of control, I'll support her.

Today's list:

> root beer
> call Dee's real estate agent re: sale of house
> underwear for Dee
> straws
> gherkins
> vanilla ice cream
> request lawyer to come to house to prepare Will and
>     house sale

Next to me on the seat of the car blinks the little green light of the car phone. It is as though I am in Intensive Care. Well, I am *intensive caring*.

## August 22nd

Dee is getting thinner and thinner. I have the phone in her room and have rerouted all business calls to other lines at her request. She feels more in control with a phone she can answer and dial, and the knowledge that I am always at the other end of it. I had provided my answering machine to spare her; but now that so much is lost, picking up the calls herself each time the phone rings is a tiny thread of attachment to the world outside, and she says she enjoys it.

Ever since our last talk on unfinished business, she's resting comfortably in her higher self. She has no inclination for anything that isn't golden smooth. No conflicts, irritations, no past, no future. She radiates.

A friend has told me about "town assistance." I've made calls, and a fat packet of applications arrives. I run up to Dee and show her.

"No way I could do that, I have stock I never told you about."

This is the woman who couldn't go for checkups for lack of money! I feel a flash of anger. Then take a deep breath, dropping the envelope into my overflowing trash bin. She is who she is. Let's see, what is next.

I need to take my granddaughter to New York to meet her mom. Rosio can only stay until two in the afternoon. I'd climb mountains for this sunshine little girl who lives so far away. So I tell Dee I'm going to get her my favorite helper, Mary, to sit with her. She's very grateful. Mary is an angel also. I haven't seen her in several years, but when I telephone, she says she will come right away in her loving Southern drawl, and I feel better just hearing it. I knew she would come. Tory and I travel to another town, meet the bus, bring Mary back to the house.

Mary takes the stairs smiling and enters the room, where she is met by Queen Victoria. Dee has turned into another person! Our grandmother was very much like this, extending a hand to any and all visitors, starting a steady flow of gracious hospitality and never-ending conversation. Dee, the shy one, is gone. She exhales, "How good of you to come. Pull up a chair."

On the train trip, I am pretty much absorbed by golden hair, radiant smile and ever-twinkling expression, always ready to transform into laughter. Tory has her Daddy's sense of humor, this little one. She puts on her walkman and alternately frowns and bursts out laughing loud enough that the man opposite us in the four-way seats is also smitten, and we all talk much of the way.

At Grand Central Station, we wait at the rotunda, she walking merrily in circles, me worrying that her Mom won't make it. Sally does show up, and I am relieved. After turning Tory over to her Mom, hugs and kisses goodbye all round. I start to cry saying goodbye to Sally, one of my favorite soul-sisters, my daughter-in -law, more my daughter-in-life I should say.

When I return at night, exhausted, hot, wishing I didn't still have the whole trip back to the bus with Mary (who doesn't drive), I find the two of them sitting in the dark, chatting and chuckling, as the sound of the train whistle blows in the distance.

"We had such a good time. Thank you for introducing us!"

This day has cost me plenty in exhaustion, stress and true currency. But the scene of the two of them together in the back bedroom talking in the darkness is one that will never leave me.

Much later, I return from Mary's bus, and say an exhausted good night to Dee. I always try to leave my irritation and fatigue at the door and just be with her. And she is so pleasant. Suddenly living the life she never quite had, she has become a person full of love, both giving and receiving, surrounded by an ideal, loving community.

I go into my bedroom where there's a single pink rose from my daughter-in-law in a vase with a pink ribbon around it. And a ceramic cup made by Tory "for Granny" in big, generous, three-year-old letters. This is a time, at last, when tears can flow, and there are plenty of them tonight.

## August 23ʳᵈ

When John is here, or the children, Sally and Tory or Jeremy and Sherry and one-year-old Ben, I am undone. There is an ancient, stuck zipper that closes when you lose a parent young. Having those you love around you for more than a day begins to unstick the zipper. We used to know a woman who cried every time she saw her doctor. I, still so young and foolish at that time, actually laughed at this and asked why. He (my ex-husband) explained, what I *should* have known; he, the doctor cared for her husband ... she had lost everyone else in the Holocaust ... one association led to another, thus the tears. Open that box and it all tumbles out. And so it is with me now. I grieve for Dee, for Mother, Father, parents-in-law, even the time I almost lost a son, all the emotion and actual losses of a lifetime, and it's hard to get that zipper back up. Old people cry *a lot*. Now I understand why.

I tell grieving clients, "Cry in the car, in the shower, at night, on Sundays. Play sad music if you have to, hut please do it for yourself." Now, I must constantly remind myself the same. Otherwise I feel I will freeze.

It is so hard. I am brick. I am steel. And then I become mush. I almost dread my loved ones coming, for what it opens in me. When our father died in 1948, the tenant-stranger, a night nurse, came and went in our home mysteriously. Our entire existence changed, yet Mother never talked about her feelings at all. This was the way Yankees dealt with life. Am I allowed to express my anguish now?

My family come to visit; and when they are here, they are totally here, but they always have to go back to somewhere else. So many friends of my age seem to be in the same situation. That was not our original vision for our "ideal lives" at all. Now, we are commuting parents and grandparents.

Three week marker. No one has mentioned chemo. I know why. Metastases are all through her. This is the horrible reason that you hear all those ads and public service reminders about "early detection." This last-minute detection reminds me of the doomsday clocks of the sixties, showing the earth running out of resources in the last three minutes of planetary lifespan. *Our* clock hands may be at two minutes to the ending.

### August 24th

Aunt Nance is the only member of the family remaining, of my generation and the one before. I feel bereft. I call her house to see how she's doing.

Wendy, her health aide, sounds very stressed. "Just a minute while I get her breathing machine hooked up." She comes back to the phone, breathing fast, and I grab her attention, an available soul mate. "Oh boy, I know how it is! How are you doing?"

"All right. But there is so much to do."

"I'm so sorry about your sister. I've been there. My mother died at Hospice just three months ago."

"I'm sorry. You must be worn out."

"I am, completely."

We have joined a secret club, the caregivers. Can anyone else truly understand? We make plans for me to come to lunch. Aunt Nance is dressing, Wendy explained, dining downstairs, and beginning to speak. Thank heavens! I had heard she could not speak and felt I had lost her. They had also said she is not to know about Dee. This made it harder for me. One relies on support desperately when on overload.

I wail to John and to the children, but this can only be done from telephones where Dee cannot hear me. This means either calls from the car, downstairs in the far offices, or in the out of town office. No one tells you that when you create a Home Hospice, your soul may be stuffed into a small box with many pigeonholes: counseling center, other office, Dee's universe.

I look forward to reconnecting with this favorite aunt of mine and also meeting this empathetic aide.

**August 25ᵗʰ**

My house has turned into an institution. Smells of mouthwash and antiseptic, schedules of visits from the nurse and the aide.

Marty now says, "She is not to go to the shower alone again. I've made that very clear to her."

They will shower and shampoo her together. This requires our larger shower. It is the only way they can both get next to her during the process. Marty has gone out and borrowed a shower seat from the Red Cross and bought a hose for the faucet. She does all these extra things to spare me, and I am so grateful.

Feeling on edge, it dawns on me that I have had a complete loss of privacy, my telephone calls, my conversations, my kitchen, now even my bathroom. Another pigeonhole in which I thought and cried, my bathroom, now has been requisitioned to Dee's world. I have no private zone remaining and no boundaries. This insight helps, and I take time to center, calm down and appreciate that I am providing what she needs. Everything else is trivial. I find a new private place inside my heart.

My personal schedule is forgotten. If I can write a check at midnight, open a book for five minutes before sleep, I just do it. And keep that list, so I don't forget anything.

> fax
> tax
> mail for Dee, ditto for me
> printer
> two clients
> groceries

**August 26ᵗʰ**

Today is my checkup. I lie flat on my back waiting for my doctor. Suddenly, I sense Mother looking down at me on the table and worrying. I tell her that Dee is in my home dying, and she sees her. She can look into the enormous house, through the nineteen rooms, into the back suite of rooms—my favorite, zero in on Dee, know the crisis with all of a mother's caring and pain. Do I actually believe this? Yes, in a way I do. When one of my sons was in critical condition, I felt her next to me. It is a moment so sad that I am crying when the doctor enters the room. It's the first place permitting letting go in days. My usually low blood pressure is up thirty points!

"It is understandable," says the sweet, Middle Eastern physician. "Not much you can do under the circumstances," he adds, really meaning it.

You can tell when they do. Personal radar works at all times, even flat on an examining table. Today, every possible resident and intern also examines me, something I have hated in the past. Today, there is no place inside me for anger. I welcome them as caregivers. Talking about my problem unceasingly, fresh eyes and words respond. It is free therapy, and I am desperate for it this morning ..

The crying opens me up for the rest of the day. I sob in the car, before my client is due and again driving home from work. I open the window and dry my tears on the highway, letting the fresh, clear breeze do the job for me. The world knows how to work very well. Just let go.

This allows me to collect myself for Dee. When I enter the room, I put aside my exhaustion and complaints and concentrate totally on her. She is pleasant, but today she had a visitor and is upset. "I couldn't open the door. Rosio had left, and I just couldn't *budge* it."

"It's never happened before." She is very critical, and I hear myself springing to my old defensiveness around her.

"From now on, just leave it open. I'd be more panicky in an emergency about them being locked out than any criminals."

We discuss EMS, "Ct. Lifeline," Visiting Nurse, 911, the doctor, my cell phone, who are all on call. She is torn. Scared of being in the house with the door open, but scared worse by what they would do for her. "I don't want to go back in the hospital. It is a torture chamber. I don't want them to put me on life support."

"I wouldn't let them. Please, don't forget we've signed the Living Will. We have it. It says no life support, even no resuscitation. I'll get some WD-40 and spray the door."

My hands shake as I wash her one dish. I'm surprised. I rarely feel the extent of the panic inside me.

## August 27th

The truth is, and we both know it, that she'll call me, ask me, and lean on me, rather than lean on any "outsider." We learned our lessons well in "codependency-dysfunctional school" as we grew up! That's one reason I am such a good therapist and she such a great nurturer of animals and people in need.

I call Hospice about support groups, as I am collapsing under the strain.

"We used to run them, but the truth is that caregivers are too busy to attend. So now, we just run the bereavement groups. People are free then, you know."

I gulp. Of course that would be so. But I could use some help right now. John is seven hours away; Aunt Nance can't talk, she is still quite aphasic; and Dee is the object of my distress, so how can I pour it all out to her? Of course not! My support system has been erased, or so it feels. Photos of children and grandchildren out where I see them helps, and I start making calls to them more frequently when I feel the worst. But I have to hunt up a time when I can speak freely, and that takes much planning. Letters to children and friends come out looking as though I am nuts.

## August 28th

Sometimes I get so full up I have to talk about what is happening, to the printer, the computer mailing-list guy, a person in a pharmacy. They have no idea what to say. Often, there is total silence. It astonishes me. Were you drowning, they might throw you a life preserver, but when the drowning is emotional, they have no way of "plugging in," unless they happen to have experienced it themselves. Their silence leaves a person breathless, when some words needed to come out. And you can tell friends, once, maybe twice, but it is a rare person indeed who makes it comfortable to discuss it a third time. I constantly ask myself, when mentioning it, how much of this is feeling sorry for myself and how much is empathy for <u>her</u>?

## August 29th

If one doesn't pin down the date, it is gone. Peel away all the petty irritations and go to the core. I have to ground the day by experiencing this core. The quality of the hours. Today it was hot, yet she was cold. I gave her an extra blanket. In the booklets Marty gave me, it says coldness is a sign that dying is underway. All the rest of life outside is just a cloud of psychic dust. It could just as well be February for all I know.

Three calls before 9 a.m., I am shaky. I decide I'll just have to put the machine on for the time before I take the phone in to her in the early mornings. The nineteen rooms, the counseling service, the training institute, the family, the entire systems that worked so well before this are simply too much on top of Dee's care. They could all fall down in an instant, like leaves off a dry branch. That's one thing death reveals. It is all a house of cards in the end.

I resolve to walk for a few minutes. If I can.

Today's list:

underpants for D.
pharmacy stuff
call insurance re: roof leak

call lawn mowing service remind to come
three client sessions
birthday gifts for Daniel, Jeremy and Tory
bank
find time to sit with her (This should be the first thing
on the list, but it is not physically possible. The things
to do are cloning themselves, running all over the pages
like ants bursting out of an anthill.)

When I get home, I feel limp.

She asks how I am, and for the first time I lose it. Words tumble out of my mouth like clothes off a shelf. "I feel as though I'm going to collapse." There I've said it. How awful. What will happen now?

"I know exactly what you mean. Once, with Mother, I felt so tired and sick, I called 911. For me. They were incredulous. They couldn't believe that it wasn't for her again. I literally had to crawl the door to let them in."

Her words are like balm. How I appreciate her understanding. We sit in the dark, listening to her ever-present radio, the sounds of the train passing through our town we loved as little girls, allowed to "sleep out" on the sleeping porch. I am at peace.

## August 30th

The lawyer came this lovely morning, in shorts and T-shirt, to handle all legal matters. What dark business on such a sunny summer day. The grass is emerald green, sunshine sparkles gold off the church tower (the one where a bullet lodged in the Revolutionary skirmishes around here), and I think of mothers and children heading for the beach with towels and pails.

I left them alone for privacy and grabbed the hour for desperately needed errands: the dry cleaners, the post office, the bank. They would be writing up a Will, disseminating the Living Will, getting her "affairs in order" legally.

What an interesting term. "In order." Emotionally, it means attending to unfinished business, old hurts, cherished memories, thank yous, goodbyes, lots of phone calls and letters. Grounding one's life by deciding who will get what. I'm glad there is time for all this. How strange it must be to know that you are on the last mile.

## August 31st

I always imagined myself taking in anyone in the family who might need care. My grandparents took in so many: cousin Shirley, so she could go to an excellent school for several years: Nelson, who lived here before being drafted and shot down over France in the Second World War, my earliest experience with stark tragedy. Then they cared for Grandfather's mother, later his widowed brother, for ten years until he remarried. That was what you did in those days. You had the space, and that was what it was <u>for</u>. My great-grandmother and both grandparents died in this house. In the sunny front bedroom, where I am sitting now. The house is full of kindly spirits; they comfort me.

The Kushi diet papers lie on the floor. The Hemlock Society's book *No Exit* has some notes stuck in it. The "Compassionate Dying" newsletter is on the end of her bed. One woman called her, but Dee chooses not to tell me the details. I ask her if she wants me to do something. I will support her in every choice.

"It's too late for all that," She says quietly. "I've stopped with the visualizations too."

In my mind's eye, I see all the little animals going round and round, like a carousel without a single rider, now stopping. We spend so much time building hope in patients. The end of hope is a giant transition, and I'm feeling a bit dizzy.

"Too panicky to put the bag over my head. Too panicky to take all those pills. I'd throw them up."

I hear you, Sister. You are me and I am you. My time is yours. My mind can contain little else. Although all the books and pamphlets remain next to you, you've done your research and decided against ending it. I don't have to have these continuing, exhausting, fantasies of calling in Kavorkian or friends who are health care providers and asking them to make themselves available to you. I have rehearsed those many times, even down to the words I would use. What a relief to let go of this question. It's been with me for weeks, ever since you said you wished you had driven into the river. Thank you for letting me release all these, like fish into a stream somewhere behind us, the memory stream of two sisters swimming together against the current, against the odds.

## September 1st

After a full day at work, I drag myself to the pharmacy because there is a message with the service that they need me to come in to pick up a prescription. A very distracted, impatient lady looks us up in her files.

"Oh, we could have delivered this if you'd only had someone call in the insurance."

How to describe these moments, when you are so worried and tired you feel like toothpaste without a tube? I want to scream, or am I just going to pass out. I sigh and say absolutely nothing. It is all I am capable of.

I hand Dee the prescription. I had called and made an appointment to talk to someone in "Bereavement" at Hospice. I just felt I had to talk. Now I cancel the appointment. There just isn't time to get to it. There has not been a time to walk, even for five minutes. I am on an emotional tether. Dee expresses no fear of death, yet she is terrified of being alone.

### September 2$^{nd}$

The children come to visit for the entire weekend. It is a great effort for them, as there are small people involved, ages one and four, as well as great distances.

"They are coming to say 'Goodbye,'" Dee says to Rosio who is sitting next to her. The starkness cuts me to the core. It seems the sicker she gets, the more direct her communication. Like a trusting small child.

When they arrive, I am thrilled and touched. The house feels whole with all this love inside it. We have meals in the dining room, little Ben spilling food out of his high chair, Tory making us all laugh. We are so full of emotion we get up and dance a circle dance with the children, and they are overjoyed. It is like "old times" when my children were little and there was so much life and laughter in their grandparents' home.

There is just one problem. Dee can't enjoy it. She can't come down to the dining room. I offer to bring people in to her room to chat, as we did in past weeks. After one marathon talk with Sally, which she loved, she sinks into exhaustion. She says, "I just can't handle it now. I am getting too tired."

This feels like her sudden, permanent retirement to her bed after she undertook the supreme effort of spraying the hornets' nest. I surmise that when you are dying, it is <u>not</u> a slow, steady decline. Instead, there are bursts when one has the will to do something very significant, and then a major collapse.

"How about one at a time?"

She shakes her head. "Can't. But leave the door ajar; I love to hear the family sounds."

As the weekend rolls toward its close, Jeremy takes matters into his own hands, slips in the room and says, "Mind if I join you?" Of course she doesn't. They have their talk. There are hugs and kisses and tears.

She sees little Ben, turning from baby to toddler, peering in through the open part of the door. This woman, who adored babies so very, very much, can't utter the invitation into the room. Ben, as shy as she once was, blows a baby kiss and waves goodbye.

## September 3$^{rd}$

The children have visited and left, and now it's just the two of us.

"Everyone came to say 'goodbye,'" she says to me over and over. She finds it so much easier to be final than I. We hear the days ticking like a time bomb. Dr. M. said two months, and one has slipped past us. We no longer discuss macrobiotic diets, visualizations, the plans we made in a daze of hope for her to make curtains or decorate her room with her pictures, photos. She really believed friends and neighbors would bring her own pretty sheets and pillowcases. She cared so much about beauty. Every inch she controlled had a plant, flowers, lovely patterns, even if they were created out of dime store paper towel or coffee tins covered with contact paper, and little seedlings growing in baby food jars. Two friends came to visit, bringing her things; the four others who she truly expected would show up because they insisted they would, never have.

I feel as though I could throttle them.

Once, when my oldest was in school, he got a horrible black eye from n a hard ball. The principal said, authoritatively, "Impossible, no hardballs in this school." I wouldn't let it rest. I summoned every ounce of will I could work up, did research, learned who <u>had</u> brought in a hard ball. How satisfying to confront the principal and be right for my boy. I wish I could think what I could do now for Dee.

One of her friends even asked me what she could send. I fell into the trap and was specific. "She'd love a pretty bed jacket." What a fool I was. Some dress up in Friend clothes, but never really are true friends. What a masquerade. It never came, and my irritation burns like a hot coal.

Now, Dee stays in the bed much of the time. The door that stayed open "so I can hear the sounds in the house" no longer matters. With the aide here, all my thoughts of a schedule have vanished. I wonder if it would have helped. In this business, there is no time to mull over much. Things happen like lightning. Rosio has brought in rye bread for "taste" and refuses to be reimbursed. The people around us all seem to turn into angels around the dying. Rosio, unfortunately, can not shop, as we'd been promised, as she has no car. No car. I was hoping so much for errand help. So be it. I'll shop. On to the next thought, moment, thing-to-do.

Each time I leave, Dee continues to ask me how long I have to be gone. It reminds me painfully of the years she never went to school, almost never went out. I had as little to do with that as I could manage. I became what some researchers now refer to as a "Superkid," lucky ones who find very early that there are neighbors, teachers, relatives who will throw out the life preservers. And we take off!

When I was seven, I rode my bike two miles to church where they made me a "princess" in the Easter pageant. Years later, Mother confessed she looked back on my childhood and felt I'd been "an orphan" in many ways. Of course I forgive her, then, and now. But when I think of how this gifted cellist, my mother, left her cello in the corner for twenty years gathering dust, while she suffered abuse and neglect, I am twice as determined to help others. I've devoted my life to that, and also never been without an orchestra for more than a year or so.

My life as an oboist may have a touch of compulsion hidden in it, but compulsion can get you through a squall. My "Superkid" subpersonality saved me from agoraphobia, codependency and so many other traps rampant in my generation. None of my children had this problem, and I am so grateful. But now I must go back, take on these ancient traps lovingly. They are parts of the legacy.

I arrange my appointments to conform to the nurse, the aide, schedules, and if I run over the time, I'm always within phone reach. I carry the portable phone wherever I go, a loving leash. Three mornings each week Rosio comes to be with her while I slip out for a few hours of clients or a stack of errands for both of us, and it's a huge relief. We've talked so often about Dee's panic that someone could not get in to save her. And her ambivalence that she doesn't want to be saved anyway. The anxiety trails behind me wherever I go. Yesterday I left the cell phone on the counter at the post office. A smiling woman ran after me with it all the way out to the car to give it to me. People can be so helpful and kind, one thing I will always keep with me from this time.

When I come home today, she's wearing the red "Do Not Resuscitate" bracelet. It stops me cold. I sit down.

"I should have driven into the river."

"Then we wouldn't have had this time in which you can be totally in charge of your dying. You've been able to plan every single thing. No shoulds. Only what you want, now."

"I know, but so much suffering, too."

I learn from this discussion that it is horrible for her. As she said, "like the flu, only ten times worse." But once again that she doesn't want to end it. Her room is still full of resource books and telephone numbers, but she is not going to do this. I let that road go. Instead I tell her, whatever she needs, I will be here.

**September 4th**

Marty brings me more books and fliers, one "For the Family of the Dying Patient." I feel deeply grateful. I may have been teaching this to many people, but never had I been through every day of a vigil with my own big sister. There is more about coldness as a sign of metabolism quitting, and now I understand why she is under two blankets while I'm still in summer clothes. I read that she will sleep more and more, and I wonder when is this is going to happen. In five minutes? In months? Will I be ready to handle it? But I know in my heart that whatever she asks I will do. It is as if a giant hand has reached down from somewhere up there and wound me like a clock. "You don't have to worry. You will do whatever is required," a voice seems to say.

"Could you just pick me up some 'STOP.' It's a home treatment dental gel." Details, details wearing me so thin I am vanishing.

"I'd be glad to."

Four drug stores. At the fifth, a giant one, they have it! I bring it home like a Christmas gift, great excitement.

"Oh dear, that's not it. Same company, same name, wrong thing."

And I'm as disappointed as a child whose little gift has been rejected on Christmas. I could cry. Once when I was about six, I made Dee a doll for the holiday, in secret. I would close my door at night and stitch away making first face, then body and clothing. She opened it up, thanked me, and that night I found it in her wastebasket. Why do such deep, deep memories have to surface at a time like this.

## September 5th

Late at night, bedtime. "I'm bleeding from the surgical site. My doctor never said *that* could happen!"

"A lot or a little?" Will we need to act fast, right now? I am wondering.

"Just a little. I think it can wait till morning."

"You sure?"

A nod, yes.

"Call if you need me. My door's always open. I can hear you easily, you know."

This is so awful. I think of Queen Elizabeth saying publicly, "It was *annis horribilis*." How I felt for that noble woman, dealing with all those divorces and disgraces from one of the most visible places to be born into on this planet, and having to make statements to the whole world.

I am finding it hard to sit still. This is a nightmare all the day, accompanied by many real nighttime ones. In the mornings, in my hypnagogic state, I wonder if it is really true. For two or three minutes,

I am unclear about what is reality, what dream fragment. I dream my ex-husband is dying, calling out for medication. Can I hurry? I dream of Dee. We are always in some strange place, and I am struggling to find her. My contact lens breaks or I lose my glasses. I can't find anyone I know. I am looking, begging, finding someone who will take us in a boat. I know from my training these are classic frustration dreams. My knowledge helps a tiny bit.

Yet in her room, the radio is always on a station she raves about. "It goes from country to jazz to folk and never stops. It's terrific!"

And I see that there still are moments of joy in the midst of this. Thank God for those moments. She has her hair set, and she is dressed on her couch. When the family visited, my granddaughter Tory was scared of the situation. She felt so much that was left unsaid. "You don't use Aunt Dee's bathroom, do you Granny?"

"No darling, why?"

She giggled with fear. "Aunt Dee is very, very old, isn't she Granny?"

I explained that Dee is very sick and I am not, and that this is not something we can catch. She was visibly relieved, but continued to remain close by me nevertheless. Her Mom, Sally, stayed in with Dee for hours. Every time she came out, we would go into some quiet room and cry. She quickly became my crying partner, but unfortunately then, every time we saw each other we would start to cry. We needed to, so badly. I think of this now and wonder where I am stashing all of those feelings, now that they are back in their caves.

This morning I hear the comedy team Nichols and May on Dee's radio, stop vacuuming, and turn it up. We both sit and listen and giggle. How we used to laugh at them, and at Bob and Ray in those old radio days. Our family never had a TV during our childhood. The radio was always on in Dee's vicinity, and thanks to her, laughter ran through our days like a bright ribbon.

## September 6th

I'm talking to my oldest son. It's his birthday next week. What would he like? He starts to answer, and there is a terrible coughing from Dee's room. This hasn't happened before. I can hear she can't end it, even with a sip of the water that's always next to her. I tell him I have to run and why and dash down the hall.

I sit next to her, while she coughs with a great deal of fear. This is something different and awful. I'm scared too. At last, it is over.

Dee gasps, "That's terrifying. I hope that isn't going to happen again. What could I do? And the pain now. It is horrible. Marty says it's the cancer eating into my ribs. What if you weren't here? What if I couldn't speak on the phone?"

"We could hook you up to the 'Connecticut Lifeline.' All you have to do is push a button. It would be on a necklace around your neck."

"I don't feel comfortable with that. I'm still afraid of what they'd do, the paramedics, when they got here. And no more hospitals. They are torture chambers."

"O.K. Let's see what Marty suggests in the morning."

I sleep with my door wide open as always, but this night I am half awake, on call as well, all the time.

## September 7th

First thing today, as I open my eyes, I call Marty and describe the coughing fit.

"Well, it's entering her lungs, and one has now collapsed. And the liver is gone, so cancerous cells will soon enter the lymph nodes, and that means great pain. I think we need to talk to the doctor and Hospice right away."

I am in emotional shock most of the day. On the way home, I suddenly realize my passport has expired and Adam is to be married in three-and-a-half weeks. I feel cheated that I haven't more than a minute to share the joy of the wedding, and I resolve to. And to share it with Dee as well. The invitations have arrived in the mail for me to send out. I hardly notice. I <u>do</u> notice I am hyperventilating.

When I come home, Rosio is looking very sad. She sits at the kitchen table.

"I think she's going to go to Hospice. She has a collapsed lung. And now she's in pain from the cancer entering the lymph nodes. She doesn't talk about it, does she?" Her black eyes look into mine.

We both start to cry now. I ask her, "How do you deal with this saying goodbye to everyone you care for?" My voice breaks as I sit down next to her at this kitchen table that I have wanted so much to be the center of Home for Dee, for us all. In the whole time Rosio has been here, we have scarcely been able to talk at all. Maybe one word of Spanish, maybe two sips of tea. As I sigh, my eyes sting with tears, asking to be allowed now.

"I do it because I lost my Mom just this way. I kind of have to. And I know I do it well."

"You are so good at it." Now I lose control of my voice.

"Most of my people have gone to Hospice. I had one real nice lady for a whole year. She went. I miss her so," her voice is breaking now, too. We are both exhausted and crying. Something has come to an end. Little Tory, her golden hair shining in a shaft of sunshine as she sits on the kitchen chair laughing with the nurse, or this wonderful aide preparing food for me on the big old stove, friends and relatives coming in with flowers and gifts and love for my sister. The radiant, home-based love, care and family time has completed itself. I see it, all sunshine and rich maroons and deep blues, like a Renaissance painting whose painter has just laid down her brush.

Some deep breaths on the stairs help me. I go into her room and sit with Dee a few moments.

"Marty says I need to go ... hospice. It's entering my lymph nodes. That's why the pain ... so much worse." She takes little breaths between words now.

"I noticed you were holding your side. You have pain right now?"

"Yes. And she says the coughing is from a collapsed lung."

"Oh my."

"I'll have to go. I can't breath right ... it wouldn't be fair to you.

She told me that Dr. M. never took out the tumor. I never <u>knew</u> that. He didn't tell me. Did he tell you?"

I feel a cold chill. Since I was not in the room when they spoke, I always assumed he <u>had</u> told her. But he, bless him, held out for hope instead.

"Yes, he did, after the operation. I didn't know he never told you."

We look into each other's eyes. There is no apology, no recrimination, just a direct gaze.

"If you'll bring me my cosmetics ... I won't need anything else."

We could have been discussing the grocery list.

"When they get the bed, I'll drive you. It's not far." (It's an hour, but I will lie all day for her if it helps at all.)

"I can't let you. I can't get dressed. I'm too weak."

I go into my room, where I lie down and call the Visiting Nurses.

Marty is out on an emergency, but the manager tells me it's all arranged and they have a bed at Hospice right now. She'll call the ambulance if I like. Psychic shock sets in. This is too fast to compute. So tired, crawling down the hall to Dee might be necessary, but this is not a day for indulgence. "Come on, walk down that hall. You can do it." An inner coach gets me moving. I sit next to Dee and ask her if she wants to go now.

"I'll have to. I can't breathe."

During the day while I was out, Dee has walked over a bridge. She has spent her last dime of energy. I can feel it in the room. How many times have I heard Bernie say that the dying "choose the moment to take their next step." And this is hers. Goodbyes have all been said, visits concluded graciously, and we have spent forty-five days together here in our "old-new" home with all the smells, memories and spirits. A gift of forty-five days. So many have none. So many without one hour. Now the time has come.

A huge, blood-red ambulance appears in the driveway. Two nice young guys in uniforms. Thank God. I need their energy and sweetness. They try to get her up but can't although she's like a tiny, emaciated sparrow.

"How are you today?" one asks gently.

"I'm dying!" she is joking, incredibly. This is how she will be with them!

They wrap her like a mummy in a winding sheet, which scares me.

"It's chilly today," the one on my right explains carefully, seeing my fear. He looks like a football player.

They carry her down the stairs. It has all been so fast I can't believe it. She walked down those stairs once to tour the house, once to make war with the wasps. And now it is all over. I want to stop the hands of the clock and scream. We talked about making curtains and hanging pictures on the walls of her room to make it really hers. We thought we had some time! "Stop! Can't you wait?" I want to scream out at God.

Going downstairs first, I glance at one of my favorite sacred views, which sustain me so here in this house. The back staircase looks out onto a beautiful balustraded porch like the ones in *Gone with the Wind*. And just beyond, a church steeple against blue sky. I intend to take strength from it. Instead, I see a strange man below approaching. Anxiety has screwed me tight today. Now I go a whole notch tighter.

Robber? Mugger? Client? I breathlessly explain to the stretcher bearers, run past them and confront him. He claims to be a client, but can't remember which counselor he has an appointment with. At the *back* of the house? I try out a few names, he says yes to one, but the anxiety stays with me as I watch him weave through the white columns of the back porch and around by the kitchen porch in the direction of the front of the building.

They set Dee down on the ground, open up the great maw of the ambulance door and put her in backwards so that I can't see her face. Dying has come between us. The whale swallows her, but I hear in her quips that she is going to befriend them, give them every drop of herself as humanly as possible, because that is who she has become. I turn away and walk back to the kitchen door. I cannot watch as the red streak of the huge ambulance backs out of the driveway.

Hospice is a new world. Far out in the countryside. Small, glowing in the night like a little space ship for people who are ready to make a trip to and beyond death. I wonder what it is like to come here, and to be so aware of this coming journey. Whoever really expects to be using Hospice? John is by my side, and I am so grateful for his presence. Inside, a front desk, a friendly looking man, a volunteer we see. It is so good that he is there to pilot us. It is a journey of terror and he is what is needed.

This is the first time there has been a "gatekeeper" between me and Dee. What a strange sensation. I have no idea what I am supposed to do right now, because I am paralyzed with emotion, but John steps in as he so often does, with masculine precision and strength. He has gotten that we are to sign in and where, and when, and all the details while I am still frozen. "TIME" and "PATIENT" I fill in the boxes with a shaking hand. The volunteer directs us to the west wing, and when we walk in the door. I am shocked to find the curtain shut all around the bed as if Dee were undergoing a procedure. Back at the house, she was wide open to all those 'family sounds,' as she put it, an inclusion of her in everything about me and the family. I ask a nurse if I can open it.

"She prefers it shut." This speaks volumes.

We enter through the curtains and talk a little while. John tells her about his trip and asks her what it is like here. A philosopher through and through, he can handle any topic with the greatest lightness and skill. Dee is so comfortable with him.

"It's nice. The woman in the next bed has a kind daughter who introduced herself, said her name is Carey. The woman behind her is dying. You can hear her death rattles. (She says this matter-of-factly.)

The doctor is very nice. He is a good friend of my Visiting Nurse, Marty, and so kind. She told me once he sat down with a patient to play chess!"

She'd like me to bring her checkbook and her stationery next visit.

"You can visit me here on days you work in New Haven."

I smile. Does she really think I will skip all the other days?

The night nurse tells her she cannot plug in her radio. "It might be dangerous." Even John can't get the nurse to relax about it. She's stern, but we keep pressing her.

Finally, she yields just a step. "We'll call the engineer in the morning."

I feel panic. Dee has left her radio on twenty-four hours a day all her adult life. "Do something to help her, my heart is beating out in Morse code." I look at her. She is not panicky. And if she were, "We have a plethora of things that help," another nurse has told me. I must keep that in mind. There is help all around us now. It is no longer just me. I suddenly feel how much tension I have been carrying and feel as though my body is made out of wood. I want to burst into tears.

Dee is surrounded by ministering angels here, and they won't do anything to intervene in the course of dying, but everything to make it comfortable and loving. I see her expression is very peaceful. What is she feeling right now? Judging by her face, an indescribable relief, as coughing and pain are now too much to endure without continuous shots and medication.

## September 8th

I bring lots of things. She thanks me. We write checks. She props the little checkbook on the eating tray, writes each entry very, very slowly in perfect little letters, enters the number of the check not only in the checkbook, but also on the bill. When all the checks come back from the bank, she'll remove them and staple them to the bills again. She could be a research scientist with her precision. (This person is related to me? A disorganized, creative, right-brain sort? Maybe we were mixed up with other babies in the newborn ward?).

Dee says she can no longer eat any food. She was nauseated all night. "They gave me shots all night for pain and for nausea."

A pleasant nurse interrupts us to give her more shots that will quiet all this once again.

"I am *so* sick of ginger ale. Could you bring some root beer and some Dr. Pepper?"

"Of course," I say automatically. The longest day of my life?

## September 9th

I try to bring a joke or funny story whenever I can. Today it's the story on the radio about the three thousand dollar cockatoo that was stolen. The thief called him the wrong name, "Rosebud," and the bird shouted, "That's not my name you idiot, my name is Harry." And that's how he was returned to his rightful owner. Dee loves these.

This afternoon she is trying to use my charge card to make long distance calls once again, but "the numbers are too tiring." To this Country Person, a phone charge card is like a futuristic invention that frightens and fascinates all at the same time. She used it many times in the hospital. I can see her disappointment in giving it up, but it's too much for her now.

"Just call collect," I hear myself saying, desperate to spare her the moment.

## September 10th

I feel I need to bring gifts. I don't have time for so many. My rational brain knows this. But it's like falling in love or having a baby. Suddenly the world changes and there is nothing but time. Or time doesn't exist at all.

## September 11<sup>th</sup>

I feel I need to bring more. This time I stop at an outlet store and buy her a shirt in the kind of pattern she would buy. She is pleased. She asks me what I plan to do about my funeral, and I realize I am not prepared to answer. I tell her I'm a bit confused at the moment about religion versus spirituality, and <u>which</u> religion, as I feel connected to three different ones. (In my heart I believe all worship the same God.) What are her thoughts?

"Please call Tel-a-phase, they were wonderful with Mother. So nice, I called them a few months ago. I'd like them."

"It was such a great idea to put the ashes in Long Island Sound where she used to go on picnics in the rowboat with her parents, that sand spit out there that you can see sticking up out of the waves."

"That was my idea." She is very proud of it.

We had collaborated on Mother's rituals with minimal discussion. I'd written the obituary, she'd handled the cremation. What a task to write obituaries for a grandmother and a mother, to chisel words so carefully out of grief, knowing it to be the last act of homage. But in those days we didn't discuss much at all. It feels so strange to be psychic twins now after all those years of passing like two ships in the night. Although, we sent out lots of signals: gifts, calls, the conveying of all family news, all-purpose 'check-ins' from time to time, during big storms, and all the ritualistic family parties on every single holiday.

We talk about the farm where we grew up, a real farm with pastures, cows, and a brook ... "Ye Tiny Inn," the shack I made for myself in the north woods out of sticks and branches inspired by Winnie The Pooh ... the kids falling into the brook every single visit ... blueberry picking, the job we shared ... plucking angora rabbits down to pink nakedness in August ... how happy Mother was to finally get back there on her retirement. In imagination, we are back there now, romping through pastures, our dogs jumping next to us with laughing expressions, drops of moisture falling off their tongues.

"The house burned. I went back to look. They made the lovely little brook into a big ugly pond. Don't go."

Her voice is getting so much weaker I have to lean over next to her head to make out the words. When she is completely drained of energy, she just asks me to put the radio back up. It's become a signal. Then we sit there, my hand on her arm, or I try to produce a monologue, which is very difficult without crying. I have never eaten here for fear of being rude as she can't eat at all now. I ask her about this. She nods, yes, do get a sandwich. With dinner from a vending machine, I sit and chew. Later we meditate, my hand on her arm. I tell her about therapeutic touch and the power of prayer.

The nurse stops me in the hall. "We need the information from your funeral home, any time you can get it." Even though I expected this completely, I am shocked.

In her book, *HeartMates*, Rhoda Levin[7] said something that touched me to the effect that, "Your cognitive skills will be shot when you are a caregiver in a crisis." I appreciate this so much tonight. Otherwise I would think I had gone brain-dead. She also wrote that, when you do your "stress management," just shoot for the things that concern you the most. This tip helps me think, when I am stuck in a molasses of tears, and fears.

### September 12th

Early today, the morning glories I planted in June suddenly burst into bloom. They point their heads up to the sunshine and seem to be responding to Dee's idea that I do something in memory of her "in the gardens," when I asked her about a memorial. I find it impossible to think of one without the spiritual. How can anyone not believe in something?

The Amish and Native Americans always left a hole for the spirit in all their creations. This is what I feel I need to do. And miraculously, I have picked up an angel that my Finnish artist friend has made out of a nut for a face and chick feathers for wings. I put this down on the tray. Dee loves it. I have chosen the right thing. And who am I to judge what is spiritual for her?

She asks me to fetch and carry a lot today. I sense she is agitated. A trip to the refrigerator for soda and crushed ice. She's asked me to check the level of the bottle that has her name on it. She is becoming obsessed with the drinks. They are all she can get down now, and she pours water and soda back and forth between various cups over and over again.

When I return, she asks the level, and I tell her. Unacceptable apparently. She shakes her head slowly, very weakly, as if to say no, and then, "Bring me the bottle."

Well, my eyes *are* terrible, and now I realize I must have seen the label and not the level. I bring the big cold bottle to her bedside. She checks it, nods, waves with her hand for me to return it.

John, who has come along today, attempts to distract us from feared tension by asking about her schooling. "Why did you stop. You had no use for their brand of wisdom?"

"Oh no! I took a guest out to the farm for the weekend, and our father passed out on top of her." She speaks like a child. Inhibitions are gone. A good combination, the Philosopher and the Little Girl. Absolute Truth today. I feel exhausted.

My inhibitions, fortunately, are not gone. I will not speak of the utter humiliation of being a little girl whose sister has vanished from school forever, and whose parents shroud secrets no one can mention in the 1950s. I lean back in my chair and just breathe. Her voice is so weak today that she asks if we could make a megaphone.

"Of course," we both say, instantly.

Back home, I call her accountant about the check she wants to mail for Adam's wedding. He offers condolences to Dee and me "for the rotten luck, and she is really too young to go. Sure, I'll put a form in the mail."

## September 13th

At hospice, there are many packages and bags. I see people unpacking them out of the trunks of their cars, trying to bring little bundles of home. I also see people bringing them back out—because their person is now dead? :Yes, kiddo, that's part of what you're supposed to learn here," I say to myself. The voice in my head has become a big help at moments when the pain is just too much. Dying involves much carrying of things. These other people seem oddly embarrassed, and I find that I am, too. Only the volunteers have not lost their tongues, thank heavens. They took me in the eye and ask how I am.

Today I feel totally alone in the cubicle behind this closed curtain. Even though I greet and am greeted by the large family that always seems to be eating, watching TV and in a big gathering to our left, nothing of this enters into the ring of dying that is our private space. A procedure is going on, and the procedure is conscious dying.

I give her the little megaphone. It is a paper cup glued inside a large plastic one. John figured it all out carefully. She handles it like a toy. Then she asks me to label it "please save." I find some masking tape and do so. "Upside down," she says and gestures for me to reverse it. She smiles raw pleasure at this gift now perfected. She is holding the shirt I brought like a baby. "It has to be prewashed," she says. "It says so on the label inside."

"I'll take it home and wash it and bring it back tomorrow."

## September 14th

Today I've brought a box of photos I've had made up for each of my sons, either upon their marriages or at age twenty-one. Adam will marry in three weeks now. (My stress points, were they gauged by a professional stress point scale, would number in the thousands. But there's no time for that.)

"You should write the identities on the backs. Now!" Dee holds up a photo and turns it over as though it were a stone. She raises her eyes at me. I notice how hard it has become for her to look at me, how heavy the lids must feel. She also has begun to gesture with a finger around the room, lacking the strength for a full hand movement of any kind. She loves the photos. She reads the wedding invitation and smiles. The room is full of flowers and cards, and the entire shelf above her is lined with exotic sodas, ginger beer, root beer, cranberry, etc.

"Marty came all the way out to see me and brought six bottles."

That would be very like Marty. Her mission is to minister to those who are hurting, and she does it with sensitivity and warmth.

A nurse enters the cubicle to give another pain shot. I've noticed Dee holding her side but there's been no further talk of pain. Not a word. When the nurse leaves, she comments, looking around, taking in the wall of cards, the row of special drinks, the flowers and plants.

"Well, you certainly are surrounded by love!"

"I have a joke." D. beckons me to lean way over so I can hear. "Two street cleaners, one points to this woman. 'She's from a very good family, her father was a school crossing guard.' I made it up myself this morning."

I think of her all the way home and how sorry I am not to have had this for the last half century and how blessed I am to have her right now. I am learning to drive in the dark, with my lousy vision and through tears.

At home, I curl up with the telephone book and start searching.

No "Tel-a-phase" in the phone book. I call information.

"Nothing at all, sorry."

She said something about California. I call their information. "Nothing, sorry. "

After a frustrating series of attempts, I am exhausted and it all comes tumbling out. "I don't know what to do. My sister is dying. She wants them for her burial and I can't locate them anywhere. Can you think of anything?"

"Of course, I'll ask my supervisor."

There is help out there. Operators are great human beings. I learned this when Sally gave birth to Tory in the hospital, and I couldn't get through for hours. When I simply told them the story, they got me through in a matter of minutes.

I thank the powers that be for this. And also for my home. When I inherited it, my grandmother had been sick for over ten years and things were in disrepair. Lampshades hung crookedly, curtains were tattered and there were smells from her beloved German shepherd. Toward the end, she couldn't control either dog or house. We once even had a Halloween party here for the children. It was the perfect haunted house. Now kids are grown with their own homes. I'm free and have cleaned, painted, restored for eighteen years. If this had to happen, this was the best time in terms of space, comfort and beauty for Dee.

### September 15th

Dee treats everyone like her best friend. Her banker, lawyer, town tax department manager, post office clerk, are all her intimates. When I take up her business now, they all say, "She was so good" or "She brought us cookies, they were delicious. She was so sweet." One man says, "Tell me if you have a memorial service. I want to be there. When she said goodbye, I could feel it really was "Goodbye."

Today Dee asked me if I could massage her legs. I guessed that she is having cramps because she hasn't stood in days now. Standing at the end of her bed, I massaged and squeezed her legs using therapeutic touch, transmitting love and healing energy as I did so. I am grateful there is something I can do for her.

### September 16th

She holds the prewashed shirt like a teddy bear next to her heart. She has slipped so far so fast, she is back to age two or three. The stuffed animals are lined up in front of her on the tray table, no longer being used for food. Some were brought from home, some sent in the mail. When I walk around finding myself a chair, fetching her crushed ice or myself a sandwich, I have taken in this place, hospice. There are many cheery events that some lucky ones get to attend because they can sit up or even talk. The weaker, bedridden, patients lie open to everyone. It is a communal experience for them.

Ours is not. We are instead totally alone, my sister's choice, much like our childhood.

Many of the dying hold big cuddly stuffed animals. Volunteers and staff come around and ask them if there is anything they can do, even though these people appear to be unconscious. It is a beautiful ritual, and I know it makes a difference. Dee has left her little animals behind, and now only clutches the shirt, her head resting against the pillow. She is becoming yellow. Her liver is going.

The letter from the accountant arrived today. It requires Dee to authorize the wedding check for Adam either on the phone or in writing. We are too late.

The drama requires many a deep breath. I've talked to my mentor, Judy, and she's had a Buddhist prayer circle praying the whole time, "either for recovery or release." In return, I must "do 52 acts of service for others," That feels like nothing these days. I know now that it's time for the release, and turn my prayers to that.

Dee can no longer use the megaphone. I can barely hear her with my ear next to her mouth. She can no longer take phone calls. She can communicate only in my ear. She is like a newborn.

The nurse tells me Elizabeth has called. Amazing, since she is starring on Broadway every night in her own one-woman show. I call her back right away so I can tell Dee.

"Oh my dear, dear friend. I'm going to put my house on the market. I don't want to ever go back to that village." A long pause. "You know, I think she was an angel! I've often thought that. I've even said it to friends."

"That's odd. Do you know she won't let me talk religion at all.

Anything of dogma, and she's very upset. But I took her this little angel my friend from Finland had made. The head is a walnut, no face, just a beautiful little head with feather wings and a white paper cone for a body, and that was just right. She keeps it in front of her all the time. And that's where the spirit is for her!"

"I'm not surprised. I <u>know</u> she is an angel."

My God is central, essential to my life. I don't know how it would be to live without holding the divine as the hub of life's wheel, every moment. I admit to confusion about religions. It feels true to me that all pray to the same mysterious force, the one that Albert Einstein found embedded in the workings of our universe. This is not a time for judging or preaching. My few references to any established religion have annoyed her. Yet when I repeatedly say, "We are all together spiritually," when speaking of the children, grandchildren and friends, she glows appreciatively.

The little angel is her favorite. This afternoon I brought her a beanbag puppy from my collection at the house, mostly my sons' childhood castoffs. As I enter the room, she points to a package from a very close friend, Vinny. I tear it open. It is another beanbag toy, a little pink one. These are sisters, these little beanbags, same concept, same size. We are certainly on the same wavelength and both know this is about all Dee can now enjoy. I line them up on her food tray along with a Snoopy I've brought attached to Halloween candy for the nurses. It is a month too soon, but there is no "time" anymore.

"That wonderful lady over there on my right. She died last night. Such a great family. Did you ask the doctor how much longer, or the nurse?"

It won't be long, I reassure her. She is becoming smaller and smaller. She looks so much like Mother that it startles me. She asked if I could bring her the photo of the two of us from the album collection that will be Adam's wedding gift. Now she has it propped up for everyone to see, the two sisters, smartly dressed up in matching winter coats and leather leggings, little girls, three and six, in clothing from long ago. She squeezes the shirt I brought like a teddy bear (prewashed and returned the next day, of course, because I too am now a hospice bag lady, bags of love, packages, bottles and mail).

Words are becoming more and more difficult. Now I meditate more, hold her hand, talk while she listens, or even bring in food. It no longer seems at all appropriate to try to be polite by not eating when she can't. Politeness is a stiff, formal, obsolete thing.

We've been so separate all these years, and now we are joined at the heart. I can't even think of losing her just now. On the way home, I think about my life, and it seems that the whole story has been about reuniting with my lost family ... all the orchestras I've played in, the organizations I've founded or joined, the networks, the clubs, the schools, all repeated efforts to rejoin a kind of family. And I wonder if that isn't true for all of us.

I meet a nurse in the hall. "How are you doing? All the arrangements made?"

So I don't have to wonder. It is coming soon. I've tracked Tel-a-phase down, and the service is no longer available on the East Coast, but they refer to selected funeral homes. They give me the names of my next-door neighbor's funeral home, whom I know, but never thought of for cremation.

I call them feeling very strange, but they greet me so professionally and warmly, all at the same time, that the visit flows smoothly. Their son used to date a friend, and he would bring me flowers. Once he said, "Today it's a child. That's really awful."

I never forgot his face, the sad expression, the determination to do right by her, the little vases of pink flowers with pink ribbon bows. We do our contracting, then engage in neighborly chat for a while.

"The body will rest here for a day or so, state law, the medical examiner's office."

I think of Dee being transported upon her death so that she will lie practically next door on this street, while we mourn her. There is something oddly cozy and symmetrical about all this.

### September 17th

I am stunned when I enter the cubicle this night. She has changed color. She is now truly completely yellow. I assume this means the end of all liver function. She whispers in my ear, and I can barely make out the words.

"I think I had a stroke last night, a very loud noise in my head, and then I couldn't see out of one eye."

I see that her right eye has turned white and try to reassure her. "TIAs are quite common. Some don't even know they've had them." (We've talked health information since we could talk at all. Born into a surgeon's home where father was up at five to operate, allowed Dee, the elder child, to color his anatomical illustrations for publications and talk surgical complications at the dinner table.)

Dee wants the bed fixed so she can breathe better. I go to the nurse's station.

"I'll get the man to fix it," the nurse responds instantly.

I go back to Dee and tell her.

"No," she frowns, "the nurse, the nurse." I sense a strong desperation in her as if she were saying, stay until she does it.

So I do. The nurse puts the head up and tries to explain to me that "way up" is *not* the best way for her to breathe, and she's "a two-person lift now." She goes and gets the second person and they lift her higher. I sense great fatigue in this nurse for the first time, and now I get it. Both the nurses and I know death is ,close and the commands are the sole remaining hold on life energy. I am close to snapping for the first time through all of this, and so are they. This is the last chapter, and we are determined to get through it with equanimity. I'm glad they told me to call the funeral home. I realize they've been preparing me without coming right out and saying so.

Tonight, Dee holds my hands in hers for a long time. It is different. And then, as always, "Thank you so much."

There is no comfort so great as doing the right thing. When it has not been done for you, there is also a deeper healing. By becoming whole, through a deliberate act of will, we close up all those deep scars within.

## September 18th

After office hours, I drive out to eat by Dee's side as I've been doing. I get a sandwich in the lonely area in the far back of the building with the vending machine and walk back through the long hallway. Nodding to the large family next to us as I always do, I pull back the curtain gently. She's unconscious. My sister, with whom I delivered puppies at dawn, ran and played in the fields in the country, hugged and cried with in the rain when Mother died. The person who's always, always been there, is lying yellow against the pillow, mouth open, eyes shut, as if waiting for something to arrive. I am so horrified that I have to walk out. In the hall, a nurse finds me.

"I called you to tell you there's been a change. I didn't want to shock you." She looks dismayed.

"I didn't check the home answering machine because I was at the office, and I had a psychotherapy client and felt I couldn't cry just then. Thank you so much." All I can do is listen to this beautiful soul as she talks, talks, while I try to locate a thought in my murky brain. There aren't any right now.

"She's been changing for two days. Believe me, I know what it's like to be trying to work as a health professional at the same time you are grieving. It's like walking a tightrope and trying not to fall off." She is talking me through trauma. Some faraway part of me knows this. One part observes, another part knows. I've been a disaster volunteer. I know about the time a person needs to "come to." I know I just need to hear, feel and think.

Finally, I find some words. "Does she know I'm here? I'm not sure what to do." I try to give myself room to breath. I guess the nurse must know about this. Of course, she does. "I think I'll just keep up my regular schedule of visits."

She looks at me. "That's perfect."

"What do you think? I do this Conscious Dying as part of my work, and we have always taught that patients know when someone who loves them is here. Would you agree with that?"

"It's not official policy or anything, but my personal view is that they feel it very deeply. I see the face when I am taking care of them, and then I see the expression when a family member is next to them. They know. I am absolutely convinced they know."

I go back into the cubicle, wondering what is going through the minds of the other three families in this room. "Cynthia, this is what hospice is all about, not hiding the steps of dying. You hear and you see the steps of dying, steps everyone needs to prepare to take. We all need so badly to know." A voice of spiritual knowing deep, deep within myself talks me through the entry back into the room, where death and the angels are waiting.

I look around the room and see, as if for the first time, the dozens of soda bottles of the special kinds she's requested for "taste," all the cards, the little toys lined up with the wooden angel in the middle, flowers, plants, all the tangible signs of love manifested in every corner of this cubicle. And now I see a huge vase of flowers on the food table where there can be no more food.

The little card dangling from this huge bouquet reads: "I brought you these, Dee, but you were sleeping, love, Carey."

Thank you, Carey, wherever you are. You came back to pick up your mother's belongings and what pain you must be feeling.

Dee is not sleeping. She is in a deep coma. Her pulse is faint, and I can't hear her breath at all. My prayers are addressed to her as a conversation, a meditation, from the place in me that I know can travel anywhere. I tell her how we are still together in spirit. How she will be with Mother and Father, our grandparents and great-grandparents, and how life is only a moment in God's eye and she will be able to help me when I come to join her. I hold her warm hand for a long time, sending energy and love, and then I put her hand down gently on the blanket.


Hospitality

Hospitable I am.
You say you are dying, I jump in the car,
drive a thousand miles to have you treated,
too late, too late, and then to drive you home.

Hospitality becomes something different.
No meals in dining rooms, nor flowers arranged in halls.
Rather, tucking you into the small back bedroom, where you
lie, thin as a sparrow, amid bouquets and cards and drinks
with straws.

Hospice, the end point.
How we'd wanted it all to unfold at home! But there comes a
time of too much pain, cells silently eating ribs, lungs
collapsing like parachutes behind enemy lines.
So one checks in to the last hotel.

Outside, there is a world of sunshine; cosmos bloom on the
garden bench.
I view my world through tears and dark glasses, looking for
my sister everywhere, finding you only in one small bluebird
greeting me back at an empty house.

# PART 2

# A COLLECTION OF THOUGHTS, QUOTES AND REFERENCES

W e had a weekly reader in first grade. It told us what we needed to know. C.S. Lewis[6] writes about death as the end stage of every love, and of course it is, because someday, in some way, we will always have to say "goodbye." But who will teach us what we need to know about <u>this</u> subject?

I created a kind of Commonplace book as I went along, the catch-all journal they used in the eighteenth century to reap the wisdom and insights of any new journey in life. It was usual in those days to make the "Grand Tour" of Europe if one were lucky enough to be able to do so. Parents sent their sons on this if they possibly could, as it was considered "essential education." Into this book, the traveler would put thoughts, sketches, visitors' cards, souvenirs and even pressed leaves. Conscious Dying may be the Grand Tour of the modern person. Today we are so insulated from death, most of us can't even discuss the topic. This is a journal about the inside and outside of death and dying.

> I cannot talk to the children about her. They look as if I
> were committing an indecency. They are longing for me
> to stop. I felt just the same after my own mother's death.
> —C.S. Lewis[6a]

Ah yes, I too felt total humiliation, returning to boarding school after being away for a week for Poppy's funeral. I remember slinking into an "evening activity," hoping no one noticed me. I was often this transparent person, and it seemed to work. At home, where pressing problems gobbled up every moment, and the problems were always sister's or father's, it was a most useful strategy. Mother was the silent one, silent except for those sighs that punctuated my childhood, and I learned to be the same. We called her "the Saint." Now I know better.

Such saintliness can kill you. Even the saints need to cry once in a while.

In the first shock of crisis, get yourself a little notebook. Then you can just write stuff down all day long. This becomes your memory, collects essentials, helps you get organized, and stores feelings and emotions for later, when you'll be longing to harvest them. My logbook was one of the most helpful things for me all those many months. When my father died, I had an English teacher who made us keep a journal. I could pour my heart out into mine, and he would write his comments in slanted red pencil. Someone was listening.

Recently, our alumni magazine asked us for memories, and I wrote this one. After it was published, he answered me. What a shining moment of connection. Ah, these are the things that count in a life.

Caregivers are overwhelmed partly because the terrain is completely unknown. If someone could only provide us with a map. But they don't. I believe the health professionals feel it would be cruel. And yet listening to others, my clients and the support group I attend as a mourner, I hear us all say how terrifying it is to witness rapid physical deterioration, to see fainting, incontinence, strokes, scars and emaciation—without having been warned at all. The professionals have been desensitized out of necessity in training, but how about the caregivers? Each condition contains its own chamber of horrors. We can't get to any kind of support session as we are too busy, and so we just shift into automatic like a car. Then we enter into the chamber of horrors: blood, collapsed lungs, coldness, color changes, inability to breath, unrelenting pain. Very much like descending stairs, and no way one can get out.

When I talked later with the others, I learned we all went through our panic and post-traumatic stress syndrome many, many weeks after the fact. If saintliness means never feeling, never talking, it's a road straight into the heart of stress. When it hits you, you've got to express something. Write, draw, call friends, keep a journal, dance and cry.

When you mention death to casual acquaintances: the man at the copying center, the pharmacist, the guy who sells you shoes (because you find, it is impossible sometimes not to tell <u>someone</u>), they simply do not acknowledge that you have said anything. Your words have fallen on deaf ears. How will they live their lives when it comes time for <u>them</u> to deal with a separation or a loss?

I sometimes drop a little note to someone or have mentioned to a social worker that I "really need to talk." Even the professionals do not respond! They are wound like tightly coiled springs to do a job and keep on doing it, no matter what. Open a letter, record something, never stop and feel. I knew this. That is why I became a trainer of such professionals. We need so desperately to unzip that stuck zipper and feel once again. Otherwise, we first burn out and then what's left becomes hard as steel.

Yesterday, one of my supervisees *had* to talk before she could discuss any cases. "I don't know what is wrong with my therapist; but I know something is. He just laughs at almost everything I say." Another burn-out symptom.

Every good therapist says, "Cry, it's essential." What they, we, don't get is that moving from here to there is not always possible. One hears or reads the suggestions, but can't move. Well, here are some composers who will get most of us started crying so you don't have to do the research yourself: Albinoni, Bach, Barber (*Adagio for Strings*), Pacabel's Canon, Hovanis. And if there's no time to shop (of, course there isn't), many public radio stations have a service where they'll order disks or cassettes for you for a small donation to their very good cause.

> ... yet H herself, dying of it, and well knowing the fact,
> said that she had lost a great deal of her old horror of
> it ... and up to a point I very nearly understood ... one
> never just meets cancer, or war, or unhappiness (or
> happiness), one only meets each hour or moment that
> comes ... one never gets the total impact of what we call
> "the thing itself," but we call it wrongly, the thing itself
> is simply all these ups and downs: the rest is an idea.
>
> C.S. Lewis[6b]

Well before this era in which we have reaped the benefits of Eastern thinking, C.S. Lewis had also stumbled upon mindfulness in his exhaustive search of spiritual literature, now the core of many workshops tending to a frazzled American public. He'd spent a lifetime delving into literature and philosophy, and wrote religious books which were solace to many. In the midst of the "thing itself" we can become truly mindful. Some of the dying do. My sister did.

All the ghosts of our fears, like the Buddhist deities at the four doors of the temple reminding us of the challenges of life, are now inside our lives, are the meditation, and there is nothing left to fear.

Steven Levine says, "If you live in an empty apartment in life, so will you in death."[9] By enriching the present moment to the fullness of its essence, we best prepare ourselves. When Dee and I breathed together, prayed together, we were joined as never before in our lives.

The great psychologist Milton Erickson discovered that having his residents go home and do psychological work with their relatives was, in fact, far more transforming than having psychotherapy! When you can spend time recalling, reliving and communicating, life smoothes out, and you can finally digest it.

When you are a caretaker, you seldom think or feel. A social worker tells me, "None of them could make the groups, too busy, so we stopped offering them."

A switch is flipped. Make a meal, shop, place that phone call, do this, that, collapse into bed at night. At times you are so dissociated you feel you are playing a part in a film. When it is over, not only do you feel the grief, you also stare into the image of what you've just been through. One woman says to me, "I would have just walked out of the room, but I thought I'd faint." Another shakes as she tells about the death of two parents within the past six months. Is there any help for this? There is, and you must try to do it for yourself! You are the only one that can say, "That's all I can take, I've got to stop for a moment." Write, even scribble in a journal. It helps unload (and raises the immune response as well)!

If you can call even one person with whom you don't have to put on "a happy face," write this on your to-do list in your notebook before you move on to the next thing, and resolve to do it. If you face burn-out from too much caring, running a home hospice, day care, care giving, even codependent relationships (i.e. if you are living someone else's life), get yourself out. It is the hardest thing of all, but you need to connect to life, talk, breathe, take in nature, for a real, healthy, vibrant, existence. One look into my garden to see the latest bloom, hear one birdsong, how they helped recover my senses!

One woman came into my office after four years of such a situation, twenty-four hours a day. Her sister had been electrocuted in front of their eighty-year-old parents. Taking care of them both in her own home, she felt she could not be emotional. She couldn't talk, think, sleep. All she needed to do was just tell me about it and cry. She cried for a year, then recovered completely.

If there is any form of Higher Power for you, the time to use it is now. The Norman Vincent Peale Center for prayer receives two thousand calls a day. We do not yet know the precise mechanism of healing and helping, but it is well documented that spirituality helps in many ways, for both the one who prays and for the prayed for. (Larry Dossey, a physician, now studies and teaches healing prayer.[4])

> Grief still feels like fear. Perhaps, more strictly, like
> suspense. Or like waiting, just hanging about, waiting
> for something to happen. It gives life a permanently
> provisional feeling. It doesn't seem worth starting
> anything. I can't settle down. I yawn, I fidget. Up til this
> I always had too little time. Now there is nothing but
> time. Almost pure time, empty successiveness.
>
> —C.S. Lewis[6c]

You might say all of the bereaved have PTSD (post-traumatic stress syndrome) to some extent. We are irritable, fidgety, distracted, off-center. A client tells me she would get in her car and end up in the wrong place. Things which seemed so important now appear meaningless.

> I was obsessed about my career. But by November, I
> noticed a relaxation in my psyche and soul. I thought
> less about what to do and more about what I was, and
> about where I felt drawn. What did others want from
> me? What gifts were being drawn out of me?
>
> —Robert Jonas[12]

In crises, I hear my inner Higher Self loud and clear. I cannot tell you if it is God, or just the part of me that holds the spiritual "juices" of love and understanding. Does it really matter? Yes, because we're all cursed with the Inner Critic jabbering. With a bit of practice, anyone can tune in to the higher voice instead, that of guidance and of inspiration. It's been recorded by writers throughout the centuries. The Psychosynthesis training helped me so much. I learned to identify the voices of my subpersonalities, like the fearful Little Sister and Superwoman, who always must achieve one more thing. My will became apparent and I could cultivate it. I learned to support and strengthen my observer and open up to the voice of my own wisdom through the higher self. Where would I have been throughout this time without that training? I can't imagine! A Home Hospice calls upon the spirit, in whatever form it may take.

Being a social worker by my first training, of course, I researched the resources, or so I thought. I called five resource people. Only two responded. I learned about town assistance, Hospice Home Care, received a fantastic dedicated hospice-trained nurse. But later learned I had missed about five other critical pieces of information because I was in shock and because we ran out of time.

So call <u>again</u>. Muster every bit of assertiveness you possibly can. If they don't call back, call once more. Become a pest. These people are paid to help you get through this! Don't apologize, ever, for what you are going through and the emotions it has created. I find most of us who become caregivers are the ones who never asked for help, rarely spoke of personal needs. If ever there were a time for assertiveness, this is it! Make notes and checklists, enlist friends and family if necessary.

My son called all over the place and sent me a huge envelope of resource material, which helped so much! Every bit of support will strengthen you. Just the receiving of knowledge and caring, even if you don't actually use it all. I couldn't have made it without our wonderful visiting nurse, our health aide, my friends and family, and a lot of prayer. There are so many moments when you have to turn it over to a higher power in order to be able to make out the thoughts in your head with some clarity, and then decipher what to do in the next moment.

Bumper sticker in New York City:

Let's put the "FUN" back in dysfunctional"

Humor certainly helps!

Whatever fools may say, the body can suffer twenty
times more than the mind. The mind has always some
power of evasion ...

C.S. Lewis[6d]

Steeped in helpfulness, a lifelong condition for "rescuers" like me, I was shocked when I prattled on to one of the nurses about how nice it was that we had had a month for conscious dying, while Dee accompanied me with something very simple about all the suffering. A moment of pure dissonance. Dee was playing a completely different tune from mine. If we truly listen to all that the dying have to say, won't we do as the Dutch do and make physicians and medications accessible if it is too much to bear for some? We do it routinely for horses, why can't we let human patients speak their truth and listen to what each tells us about his or her unique experience? One bereavement counselor seems befuddled and just says to call her if we'd like to talk. Neither of us will, I assume. Yankees to the core.

My grandmother smiled peacefully after a lengthy visit with the family and said, "Isn't this a lovely house," less than three hours before her death. I can still see her reaching out for my baby's toes and holding them so lovingly. My mother, on the other hand, was in agony from emphysema, and the morphine shots did not cover the prescribed time periods. She said it felt like a knife in her lungs. I ran to the nurses' station and begged them to bring the next shot. I called hospice way back then and got the kind medical director, who found us a doctor in the right town who would take away those dreadful time limit prescriptions. Just as another had agreed on that earlier fateful day when we met in Danbury to her clearly spoken wish to "discontinue treatment." We individualize toddlers in nursery school. Why not wise ones who are living a final chapter we need desperately to learn about? Listen to the patient. Each experience is unique.

There is assistance: Compassionate Dying, The Hemlock Society, books by Steven Levine,[9] Elizabeth Kubler-Ross, Kavorkian's phone number for those who want it. Even an hour of research can help immeasurably.[3]

> But Oh God, tenderly, tenderly. Already month by
> month and week by week you broke her body on the
> wheel whilst she still wore it. Is it not yet enough?
>
> —C.S. Lewis[6e]

This is the hardest part of all, the "breaking of the body." You resolve to do whatever the patient needs, out of love. What you don't know is that she will start to strangle on her own coughs late at night, when the two of you are alone. Or that her mouth will feel very "funny" to her, and she will pull strange-looking things out of it while you are talking because she has lost judgment. She will ask you if the nausea is better, when it is <u>her</u> sensation., not yours. She has lost the "healthy boundaries" we therapists know are a sign of normal development. We have merged. Our egos are connected. (It's only a mouth fungus, but how were we to know? I've spent a lifetime around doctors and worked in hospitals for years, but when we caregivers sit and talk later we all share that the physical devastation is one of the very worst parts.) Each week you wonder what horrendous surprise is in store for you next.

In cancer, someone seems to have put the film on fast-forward. So many in the bereavement group have lost someone, ostensibly healthy, in the space of a month or two. The impact on us is devastating. We can't see the world as we used to. I have to feel our purpose is to help people learn to use every day, every hour, to make this world a better place. And I think we should make war, nationally, on cancer.

Morrie Schwartz talks with Ted Koppel in a long (PBS) video on his experiences dying. He has interviewed his nurse and knows that the swallowing, the talking, and the breathing will all go at about the same time. Good for him, and for her! What a smart and wise man, this Morrie. If a caregiver could have a little sheet of what may be expected with a particular diagnosis, how merciful that would be!

Partial leads to get you started:

Social Services can tell you about after-care places for those who have no caregiver, or the visiting nurse and home health aides for those who <u>can</u> be in the home.

The doctor will tell you the overall future picture, but this may require you being quite assertive and precise in your questions. They want so much to <u>spare</u> us. That's why they are doctors!

Nurses hold the secrets of the day-by-day. But even they are too kind to lay it all out. I found the most precise information of all in the written materials I located on the specific illness. These are available from many health organizations, the Visiting Nurse Association, public libraries and on-line.

Empowerment is one answer. This is why those of us who work with this have a big bundle of resources. We can't do it for a person, but we can keep giving them little gifts of power; a phone number, an 800 number for a packet of alternative and traditional resources, a place for wigs and scarves, a new herb for nausea. And always, we do not prescribe. We say you have the information. You choose from among it all and don't stop your conventional treatment.

> Indeed it was something ( almost) better than memory.
> An instantaneous, unanswerable impression. To say it
> was a meeting would be going too far ... Yet there was
> that in it which tempts one to USE those words.
>
> —C.S. Lewis[6f]

Almost all of us who share impressions find that we have had these vivid moments after they are gone. Almost seeing them, certainly feeling their presence. Once, when my father-in-law was less than a week dead, the housekeeper's daughter came into the kitchen and said, "Why is that man praying in the comer of the study?" She was just three at the time. Her mother went in and saw him as well, in the very spot he had always said his morning prayers.

When I rushed to the hospital when my son was in a life-threatening crisis, I felt Mother sitting next to me in the car. It was a visceral warming.

Many of the group members have signs or intense longings for signs to share. We seem to feel abandoned and betrayed after all of our superhuman efforts, and a sign would be an indication we are not forgotten. They've found the same to be true of most bereaved, in research studies of widows in England. A significant number saw or heard the deceased in the weeks following death. Is this the brain's miraculous way of sending comfort to us? Or can we communicate with the other side in some as yet unknown way. There are now studies showing how dogs and masters can communicate across huge distances, suggesting that knowledge of someone close to you dying or other telepathic communication is not just anecdotal.

Many have said of the near death experience reports, now numbering in the thousands, that these are also just the biochemistry of a brain shutting down. Could it not also be a very thin veil between life and death, which can be crossed far more easily than we know yet? The esoteric and metaphysical traditions have taught the latter for thousands of years. With the new physics, we learn that everything is in fact one fabric. How do we know communication isn't a part of it?

Other group members keep asking for a sign. Many professionals would dub this "magical thinking," yet the highly respected C.G. Jung reported synchronicities regularly in his patients. People having a Psychosynthesis, doing deep personal and spiritual work, do as well. This week one woman tells me of her dilemma of indecision in taking her next step, coming out of her bereavement gradually, and how once she decided to do this particular thing, she experienced hearing chimes three times in one week! Once on Christmas, once in a store and, finally, in her brand new apartment, left by mistake by the previous tenant! "Chimes have been my symbolic connection to my mother ever since her death."

> I think I am beginning to understand why grief feels
> like suspense. It comes from the suspension of so many
> impulses that had become habitual. Thought after
> thought, feeling after feeling, action after action.
>
> —C.S. Lewis[6g]

> Bereavement is a universal and integral part of our
> experience of love.
>
> —C.S. Lewis[6h]

An admirable program. Unfortunately it can't be carried out. Tonight all the hells of young grief have opened again; the mad words, the bitter resentments, the fluttering in the stomach, the nightmare unreality, the wallowed-in tears. For in grief, nothing 'stays put.' One

keeps on emerging from a phase, but it always recurs.
Round and round. Everything repeats. Am I going in
circles, or dare I hope I am on a spiral?

—C.S.Lewis[6i]

I thought I could describe a state, make a map of sorrow.
Sorrow, however, turns out to be not a state but a
process. It needs not a map but a history, and if I don't
stop writing that history at some quite arbitrary point,
no reason why I should ever stop. There is something
new to be chronicled every day. Grief is like a long
valley ...

—C.S. Lewis[6j]

How long does one attend a group? People often ask this. One
girl is back a year later. "I lost my mother more than a year ago. But my
life is still on hold."

Returning to the group I attend, over coffee, I bump into the man
who sat with his dying wife opposite our little cubicle, while Dee and I
were at hospice. For all the hellos and goodbyes, the cheery accessories
of social relating, we have never before looked into each other's eyes. He
can hardly speak. "Wasn't that terrible! It was so horrible. I still come
by every night with donuts for the volunteers here. I don't know what
else to do. And the last day. That has to be the worst thing you've ever
gone through."

He has seen me enter the cubicle. Leave the cubicle. Reenter. He
has, in a sense, been with me the whole time. We have a bond so deep
words cannot be found for it. I remember the words of C.S. Lewis, to the
effect it just keeps going round and round. It is true of all of life. We are
who we are, and we keep walking up a spiral staircase. And we'll meet
the same sorrows, the same odd quirks of personality, so long as we
climb the climb of living. At the same time, newness is always entering.

There are partial recurrences, but the sequence doesn't repeat. Here, for instance, is a new phase ... I have been revisiting old haunts ... And this time, the face of nature was not emptied of its beauty ... on the contrary, every horizon, every clump of trees, summoned me into a past kind of happiness, my pre-H. happiness.

—C.S. Lewis note[6k]

I'll often tell a client who is carrying a load of old pain; Watch what comes into your life. Every person, place, thing. I myself read every book someone tells me about personally. Watch for the synchronicity of words recurring or themes, like the woman whose symbol was the chimes. If you watch, keep your eyes open psychically, log in your journal, the way becomes so much easier. Jung made the discovery when his patient spoke about scarabs, and a scarab-like beetle flew in the open window of his office just at that moment. This is one of the gifts of modern psychology.

I took my youngest and his wife on a tour of our "memory lane." Now married six months, they came home to me for a visit. We went back to find the old farm, and although much is changed, there was a great joy in the finding of it, in discovering tiny seedlings planted in childhood are now giant evergreen trees in the sky, that the yellow reeds rise tall next to the old brook, hollowed out into a pond, but the waters still rushing through to tomorrows. Going back with someone you love and trust to old times, being able to talk the truth and cry, is so healing. I can't put words to the new level of relaxation we reach together.

My jottings show something of the process, but not so much as I'd hoped. There was no sudden, striking, emotional transition. Like the warming of a room or the coming of daylight. When you first notice them they have already been going on for some time.

—C.S. Lewis[61]

At Aunt Nance's for lunch, I almost break down as I start to say, "It was quite a summer." Then, feeling for her, I catch it, like a hiccup, and breathe it back in. We speak calmly, dispassionately of Dee's death. My aunt can share her criticisms of Dee, all valid, one has to admit. I couldn't do this. I know I couldn't. Yet listening, nodding, helps me.

"She knew for months, Darling, that she was sick. I drove her to the medical research library repeatedly. But she did nothing!"

Not knowing what to say, I just sit and nod, and share the lovely lunch of consommé and an herb omelet her aide has prepared. We sit in the splendid garden room, surrounded by Chinese porcelain jars with shiny dark plants that look practically polished. Her home has always been perfection, as if she had floated out of some magazine illustration. She looks at me with wisdom far beyond even her eight decades, and I recall her recent confession to me, "I am also a seeker."

"Well, now you can relax. There's nothing more to be done."

I can't quite hear or believe this. It feels as if there is so much to be done. It feels like chasing ambulances, putting in tracheotomies, calling nurses and doctors, doing brain surgery. My deepest phantasmagoric images an eternal emergency room. These are the stuff of my nightly dreamings. But she's right. My devotional tasks are now mainly getting forms notarized and into the mail. I'm incredulous. She is <u>right</u>! Will someone inform my pounding heart?

> Praise is the element of love which always has some joy
> in it. Praise in due order; of Him as the giver, of her as
> the gift.
>
> —C.S. Lewis[6m]

My family always spoke loud and clear, almost proudly, of their lack of religion. I was born different, perhaps from another planet? When a little girl, I used to sit on a rock filled with mica, chips reflecting the sun, and talk to God. I knew this was a topic they all resisted strenuously. Yet now, when John and I attend a traditional mass on Easter, I find, to my surprise, the presence of all three of them among the incense and the lilies.

Months later, another concert in a church in a different state, the red rose coloring in the stained glass window is cheering. Tuberous begonias in straw baskets warm the pews. The harp vibrates ethereal music through the rows of listeners. And once again my spirits return for a visit. One of my clients found this peaceful inner connection at graveside. Another by *talking* to her dead parents for a few months. Man cannot live without spirit. Each time a culture throws it out, it resurfaces in yet a new guise. Why don't we just give up thinking we can handle it all without this numinous force? Edgar Mitchell, standing on the moon, was so awed that he established the Noetic Society upon his return to earth. And the Noetic Society has catalogued hundreds of cases of spontaneous healings and remissions, remote viewings, and other mysteries.

There is a time it will hit you, and you will be utterly exhausted. Exhausted beyond words. Let it be. Let rest come in and cover you with its healing warmth. Perhaps you'll start with just an hour. Practice. Make it an hour and a half. Three. A half day. An entire day off. Call it stress management if you need to, but take it.

What is taking me so long? I keep thinking I should not be so mired down in exhaustion and confusion. I tell myself it is time to plant the garden, to write poetry again, to put photos into books, and answer letters. I forgot that the rhythm of healing and change has its own time. What's taking so long? Life.

And then there's the guilt, beneath everything you do. All survivors must wrestle with how it is that <u>you</u> are here and he or she is not. Do not allow it to close your heart. Check it from time to time. If it has closed again, gently work with yourself, write in the journal, meditate, pray, do body work, healing touch, spiritual practice. Who knows the number of our days, or how, or why? You must wrap up the guilt and toss it away, far, far behind you.

There is life to be lived for self and others loved and loving, past, present and future. Move into your future now, honoring your open heart. The greatest blessing is to be able to manifest love through care.

Who knows the number of our days, or how, or why? You must wrap up the guilt and toss it away, far, far behind you. There is life to be lived for self and all others loved and loving, past, present and future. Move into your future now, honoring your caring. The greatest blessing is to be able to manifest love through care.

> The temple bell stops
> but the sound keeps coming
> out of the flowers

> Zen Haiku Master Basho
> —*Awakening the Buddha Within: Lama Surya Das*

# NOTES

1. Bernie Siegel MD, has become internationally known as a physician-healer, who had the precognitive genius to talk about a number of roads to strength, hope and healing, years before they were fashionable. I first met Bernie when someone very close to me had a "terminal": ("so-called" diagnosis, because this often is found to actually NOT be true and this turned out to be the case years later) and refused any of these ways of proceeding. I was so distraught I called Bernie. As was his custom, he saw me at no charge and gave of himself one hundred percent.

That was over fifteen years ago. This past year, when fundraising for local public television, he insisted on using his break times to call people back who needed support. So it is still the very same Bernie! Among his books are: *Love, Medicine and Miracles*, Harper and Row, NY, 1986; *Peace, Love and Healing*, Harper and Row, NY, 1989.

2. Synchronicities—a term coined by Jung, who observed that when we are doing spiritual work on ourselves, we tend to have a number of coincidences that cannot be explained by cause, or in any rational way, which all relate to images and ideas about our mission or purpose. I have had so many synchronicities since 1978, my pivotal year, I could write an entire book just about them. Since the day I met Bernie, our lives have been braided together in a way that no one could ever explain. There have also been synchronicities with other people, with symbols, and activities. Another time, I went to a workshop on "imagery and play," where I created a symbolic drawing, and less than one week later one of my soulmates led me to a woman who gave me a necklace with this exact shape as its pendant. If you are open, you will come across many stories of synchronicities.

3. What is a "Bernie Siegel" type? Or a Stephen Levine, Elizabeth Kubler-Ross, Carl Simonton type? A health professional who has been "called" to listen carefully, hear the unique experience and wishes of a patient or family member and respond appropriately on the spot. At the present time, we are blessed with thousands more. We train doctors and nurses through Exceptional Cancer

Patients, and books and talks by doctors like Leo Frangiopane, Patch Adams, and so many others are all contributing to this work.

4. Research on prayer is abundant now. My favorite is the study at Southern California Medical School in which cardiac patients were divided into two groups after surgery. No one knew which group was prayed for. The prayed-for group did significantly better. Larry Dossey MD is now giving workshops on the efficacy of prayer all over the country.

5. 3-D was the latest thing when we were children. You were given special glasses to wear at the movies for a greater sense of depth. Our knowledge of the Second World War was amazingly superficial, apart from this incident of the "mad woman next door." Our parents listened to the news but never, ever, discussed it. Many troubled families have little awareness of what's on the news or even in the neighborhood. When their children grow up, this makes for self-centered people, but like everything else, this disability, too, can be transformed through work and will.

6. C.S. Lewis, *A Grief Observed*, Bantam Books, NY, 1976

   6a p.67
   6b pp.12-13
   6c p.47
   6d p.1
   6e p. 47
   6f p.23
   6g p. 52
   6h p. 55
   6i p.67
   6j p.68-9
   6k p.20
   6l p.71
   6m p.72

7. Rhoda Levin, *HeartMates*, Prentice Hall, pub. 1987. This is a book that you can actually read while in crisis. She has distilled the wisdom of transpersonal therapy and Psychosynthesis with the life experiences of a cardiac spouse and trained social worker. Her suggestions help immediately.

8. Carl Simonton, Stephanie Matthews-Simonton, *Getting Well Again*, Bantam Books, NY, 1981.

9. Steven Levine, *A Gradual Awakening*, Anchor Doubleday, 1979; *Who Dies?*, Anchor Doubleday, 1982.

10. In Psychosynthesis, you are taught how to work with subpersonalities. Subpersonalities are natural clusters of needs, feelings and traits, found within everyone's personality. We work with them to speed up our progress in life and meet more of our goals in terms of personal meaning and purpose. They are fun to observe and appreciate and can bring about profound change. If you'd like to work with yours, you can read more about them in *What We May Be* by Piero Ferrucci (J.P. Tarcher).

Subpersonalities are called "alters" in the diagnosis called "multiple personality," which has gotten increased attention lately. What a "multiple" is completely unaware of, the rest of us can observe and direct, namely the cooperation of different parts (like the "wimp" and the "strong one"). This is valuable.

When someone is thrown by an illness, many can develop an inspired "winner-survivor" subpersonality that is able to summon up energy and direction and even in many cases overcome symptoms. If you are a person who disorganizes when you go inside your imagination, do this work outside, through drawings, psychodrama, cartoons, even paper dolls or mobiles. For a more academic discussion, Cynthia P. Russell, *Diagnosis* in: Proceedings, International Psychosynthesis Conference, August, 1997, San Diego, CA. For work with the Psychosynthesis concept of the Will, I highly recommend *The Human Patient*, by Rachel (published under) Naomi Ramen MD, Anchor Doubleday, Garden City, NY, 1980.

11. James Pennebacker has shown that keeping a journal actually raises the immune response.

12. Robert A. Jonas, *Rebecca. A Father's Journey from Grief to Gratitude*, Crossroad Publishing, 1996.

# WAYS TO CLARIFY AND CENTER

In what follows, there are some ways to clarify and center. Keep your work very simple and light. Let yourself be playful. Keep a book of your sketches and ideas, but don't let a perfectionistic part of you take over.

After all aspects of this work, it is valuable to leave a space in your life to digest the lesson. Try not to rush into new material or activities before you've allowed yourself to do this.

## The Evening Review

Studying Eastern systems of mastery and spiritual practice, Assagioli came upon Yogic ways of stilling the mind and learning from life. This practice is thousands of years old.

Sit quietly at the end of the day and close your eyes. Very slowly, as if there were a VCR in front of you, switch on a black and white film of your life the last twenty-four hours.

As if you could rewind very, very mindfully, play one hour at a time, backwards, until you are all the way back at the same time a day ago.

Example:

I noticed that during dinner all I could think about was him. I was not hungry and had no sense of taste.

All afternoon I was sleepy, but after meditating, my energy carne back. I would like to give it more time when I can.

Busy morning as usual. But compassion came more easily this day.

When I got up in the early morning, I was grateful that I had laid my clothes out last night. I was too crazed to plan what to wear.

As I awoke, hearing the birds singing in the tree outside my window, I turned to prayer.

When finished, digest what has happened during this experience. Take time. Write in a journal what you have learned this day. Plan grounding steps for changes you like to make. See Assagioli and Ferrucci hooks in Refs.

## Disidentification

Many therapies and groups teach us to "let go and let God," turning our problems over to a Higher Power. The 12-step movement talks a lot about "detaching."

In Psychosynthesis we have an earlier step that we practice, which enables us to let go and move up more easily.

Disidentification allows us to move back, center and re-choose. Assagioli writes in his books of how we can be clear that we are not our body, our thoughts or even our problems. We are a clear center of awareness.

Even those in pain or going through extreme stress can learn to shift to this center of consciousness.

After a day of caring for my sister, running too many errands and then meeting a new problem as I walked in the door, I could slow my breathing, return to my center, go to a quiet place inside me and disidentify.

Consider an issue in your life today. Then look at "all about that" in your mind's eye and realize that that is there, and you are here.

Make a conscious choice to leave that there. Coming back to the pure center of your awareness, continue to choose to be centered and clear. From this place, you can meditate, work on a issue with guided imagery or shift to your Higher Self and focus on inspiration, meditation, or receptive meditation.

It fascinates me that our culture now has come up with a new expression, "Let's not go there," which wards off excursions in conversation that might be come troubling. This is related to the practice described here.

## The Ideal Model

Joseph Campbell is well known from the rich series on PBS with Bill Moyers, *The Power of Myth.* I have learned much from his speaking and writing. One such concept is *Indira's web*, an Indian image of the fisherman's net, pulled out from the sea, full of flotsam and jetsam, everything from an old shoe to a piece of gold.

You can consider the Indira's web of your life. In mine, I find papers I no longer need to keep; a new friend, like a piece of gold to me now; all the other aspects of my life, work, play, relationships, finances, writing, workshops past and future. It is very helpful to imagine this in detail as a meditation and then draw it. Every time you do this, you will find changes and surprises.

Roberto Assagioli teaches *the Ideal* in Psychosynthesis. Building on the knowledge that we can increase motivation by vividly imagining our desired outcome in any area of living from fitness to completing a book, he takes his readers step by step through the process, as we trainers do our students.

You can build an Ideal Model for your life. Imagine what you would like your life to be three or five years from now. Who would you be with? What is your work? What is your play? Where do you live? What is the greatest source of satisfaction to you?

When you have reflected deeply on your meditation, plan a step to ground what you have discovered. (Grounding refers to actualizing your work with an action plan before it starts to fade.) For example, if you really yearn to create a statue, a first step might be just buying the first piece of stone to work on, or taking a class.

## The Will

Rarely in this culture do we hear about "Will." I certainly had a strong one, going to a school where we hiked a mile to breakfast in subfreezing temperatures, dumped the garbage and cleaned the cow barns. (We all had a great time!) I had a developed one, when I took up music and practiced after breakfast every morning for years.

Aside from the Arts or serious athletics, I had little awareness of will. With his synthesizing mind, Assagioli studied Eastern practice and disciplines, as well as ten or twelve other fields. In his books you can find many discussions of the Will, as his genius pulled it all together, and how to strengthen and refine yours.

A quick and easy way to start for your purposes now would be just to review your caregiving role, or any other role you play that requires dedication and constancy.

Take a few days and do a review of them. Like a scientist, explore what it is that you do when you pick up the commitment again and again. What do you do when you are tired? How do you help yourself reconnect? How does it feel?

After meditating on your personal Will as it manifests in your life right now, imagine that you are standing in a lovely garden in the sunshine and have two choices laid out before you. Consider one possible decision for a while, then reflect upon the experience. Now choose the alternative, following the same steps. When you feel you have completed this exercise, choose one and plan and record a grounding step.

When I decided to make my house more livable, my first grounding step was to spend time in each of its many rooms. Then I grounded my experiences by sketching ideas for each in my journal.

A journey of a thousand miles begins with but a single step.

—Lao Tse

This place of the squeeze is the very point in our meditation and in our lives where we can really learn something. The very point where we are not able to take it, or leave it, where we are caught between a rock and a hard place, caught with both the upliftedness of our ideas and the rawness of what's happening in front of our eyes—that is indeed a very fruitful place.

—Pema Chodren, Shambala

# THE PATIENT AS TEACHER PROGRAM

My work in this area probably officially began when I read the thesis on "Iatrogenicity in a large Medical Center." Why, one has to wonder, was it left on my desk? I was the lowest of the low, a brand new medical social worker, waiting for referrals in a brand new role.

Whatever the reason, it <u>took</u>, and I've been concerned about patients ever since. My son's horrendous experience with complications, and following near disability, were life-changing experiences. To call out for help and have no one respond when your child cannot take a breath is never to be forgotten. This sensitized me for life, so that when my mother was in the hospital and they misplaced her four times, or later in the nursing home when the morphine shots were inadequate for her excruciating pain, I began to start seriously observing these situations with a purpose, trying to sensitize people "on both sides of the desk" to prevent them.

For the peak of the research, I gathered four other women writers and professionals, and we met almost monthly for several years as a "think tank." As we became clearer on our specific focus, we invited speakers join us—a hospital chaplain, a patient advocate, others—and also went to visit and interview health professionals such as Bernie Siegel, local nurses, doctors, technologists. Our carefully designed questionnaire was administered to dozens of people at workshops locally and nationally, at speaking engagements, by mail. One woman even sent audiotape from California describing her ordeal following stomach stapling surgery.

Our research team has disbanded, but I continue to solicit and analyze descriptions of what patients appreciate or object to most while undergoing diagnosis or treatment. We have compiled a lengthy report on the research that we plan to publish. In the meantime, I present this work internationally, nationally and locally, and it has been excerpted on-line by the Yale Medical School "Humanities in Medicine" program.

# ACKNOWLEDGMENTS

L ike a lightning strike, this came down out of the blue. Did Dee have any inklings? I certainly did not.

    I don't think I could have completed this painful journey without the help of my friend John Ciampa. This time, he served as Command Central while I was journeying back from California, and then helped me think and prepare for Dee's imminent arrival in a very disreputable suite of rooms and wend my way through some of the saddest days that followed.

    The Psychosynthesis community supported me so much. One said, "We are your family, Cynthia," and it is true. Marilyn Acquarula, Gus Morrelli and Anne Ziff offered advice, suggestions and presence.

    The hospice teams, both in hospice itself and the hospice-trained nurses in our own town, were there for us as soon as we connected. Dee's attorney, Thomas Weldy, did far more than was essential, out of his sensitivity and caring. My training and friendship with Bernie Siegel MD were so valuable in getting through the daily process it is hard to imagine what this would have been without his influence.

    I thank my family, Shirley Dawson and the West Coast tribe, my ex-husband Jonathan, Daniel, Jeremy, Sherry and Ben, Adam, Sally and Tory, for their visits and supporting love for Dee and me. Elizabeth Perry and Vinny Meeks for standing by throughout our ordeal and never burning out.

    May they all reap the rewards of their compassion.

www.ingramcontent.com/pod-product-compliance
Lightning Source LLC
Chambersburg PA
CBHW031139090426
42738CB00008B/1152